# Dr. Wright's
# How am I?
## Guide

by
C Michael Wright, MD

with illustrations by
Quincy Bock Stokes

# Contents

## Section 4: Brain and Mind Health

## Section 5: General Advice and Conclusions

# How am I?

If you are feeling older by the day, and in search of a concise guide to help you navigate the most common health issues that your future may hold, then this book is designed for you. Conceived and written by a preventive medicine expert, the format consists of questions and answers about the most important medical problems we face. Youth confers maximum protection from disease. Our immune systems are primed to defeat invading organisms. Our tissues can heal quickly and efficiently. Wayward cells that might turn into cancers are targeted for removal. But once we reach 40, tissues start to lose their resilience. It's time to learn a little more about what can go wrong and what we can do about it.

How easy is it for non-medical people to gain a basic understanding of the conditions that promote disease and the actions that can forestall or prevent disease? Certainly there are many books on preventing heart disease, cancer and other chronic conditions. There is also the vast digital content of the internet that can be explored with appropriate search words. This guide, on the other hand, is for those who would like to have concise, understandable descriptions of complex subjects, distilled into a visually pleasing format. We do not pretend to provide exhaustive descriptions of all the problems that surface like crocodiles in the muddy waters of our advancing years. Instead, we offer brevity and clarity. This handy guide gives readers a tour of the main threats of aging, with an emphasis on practical, actionable information.

So consider this book a companion in a journey towards a better future. If you can master its contents then you will have -

- a foundation for interacting intelligently with your healthcare providers
- the knowledge for actively improving your lifestyle choices

A little knowledge can go a long way. When it comes to your health, myriad daily choices produce metabolic and physiologic changes that accumulate over months and years. It's never too late to start taking better care of yourself. You now have in your hands the core knowledge required for successful aging. It's up to you to apply it and reap the benefits!

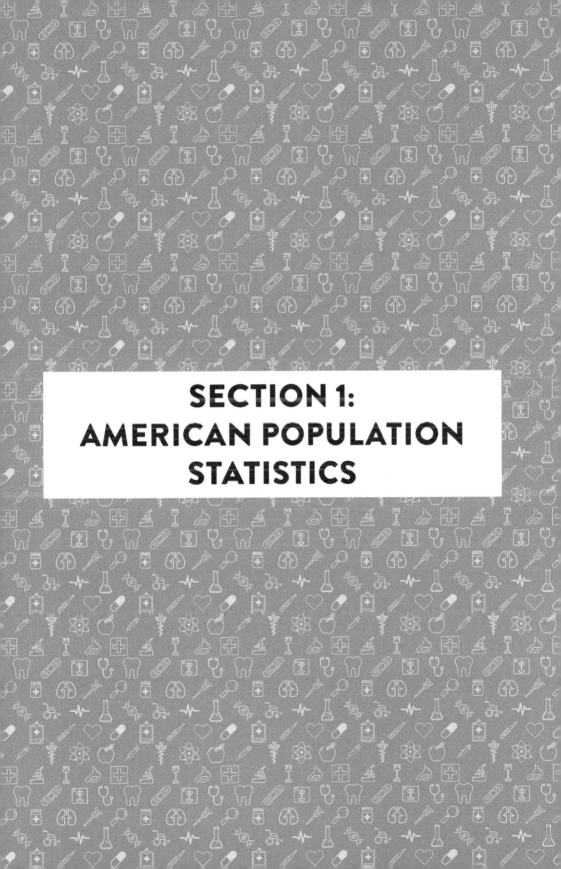

# SECTION 1:
# AMERICAN POPULATION STATISTICS

# How healthy is America?

Before we dive into the question "How am I?", let's consider briefly the question "How are we?", where "we" is the population of the United States. If we are less healthy as a whole than the citizens of comparable wealthy countries, then it means that there are most likely significant environmental and social forces at work that make it harder for an American to remain free of chronic disease. Sadly, Americans are much less healthy than the citizens of other developed countries. One way of looking at this is with a comparison of deaths per 100,000. The following graph compares Americans to 16 other developed countries, for rates of non-communicable diseases. As can be seen we are almost in last place!

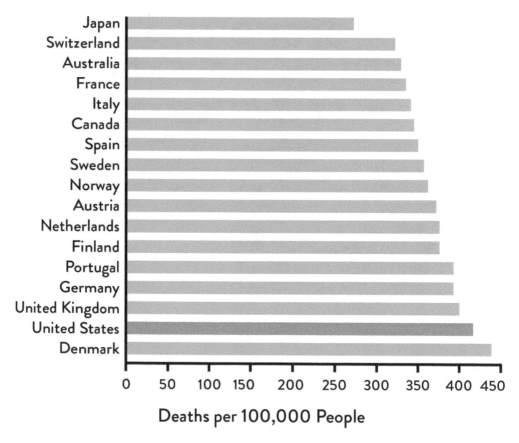

Deaths per 100,000 People

4

Japan's death rate is about 40% less than ours, and many European countries have rates that are 25% below ours. This means that when each country is standardized to a similar population range across age groups, the death rates are much worse in America. What can explain this? There is no simple answer. The American lifestyle is more sedentary, with a greater dependence on cars. It is more individualistic, with less taxes directed towards healthcare, education and other social programs. The American diet is not as strongly rooted in traditional cuisines, and Americans use more processed foods and fast foods. America has more obesity that most countries. To help answer this question, researchers in England published a study in the Journal of the American Medical Association. They concluded:

*"Based on self-reported illnesses and biological markers of disease, US residents are much less healthy than their English counterparts and these differences exist at all points of the socio-economic status distribution."*

Even though England is just slightly better than America in the standardized death rates comparison shown above, its population is significantly healthier than ours. The authors of the paper found that diabetes rates were 12.5% in America vs. 6.1% in Great Britain. For hypertension the rates were 42% vs. 33%; for stroke, 3.8% vs. 2.3%; for cancer 9.5% vs. 5.5%; and for all heart disease 15.1% vs. 9.6%.

The researchers drilled down further to look at various biomarkers for disease. Biomarkers are used to predict risk for future disease. Abnormal level are associated with a perturbed metabolic state. Over many years, these metabolic abnormalities increase risk for chronic diseases such as cardiovascular disease and cancer.

For example, C-reactive protein and fibrinogen are both molecules measured in the blood that are linked to an inflammatory state. Higher than normal levels are predictive of a higher risk for cardiovascular disease. In the British study, both of these biomarkers were significantly higher in Americans than in the British group. Many aspects of the American lifestyle, including higher stress levels, sedentary lifestyle, poor nutrition and obesity, are associated with low grade chronic inflammation.

The British study also found higher levels of HDL cholesterol in Brits compared to Americans. HDL cholesterol is protective, with higher levels associated with lower risk for heart attacks and strokes. All the same lifestyle conditions mentioned above are also associated with low HDL cholesterol.

So when we ask "How are we?", the answer is clearly that we are sicker and die younger than people in other advanced countries. One well-known study tracked the risk for heart attacks in Japanese that had moved to America. Rates of heart attack are very low in Japan. But after migrating to America, within one generation their rates were similar to those of Americans.

When people come through the Scripps Center for Executive Health we focus closely on biomarkers and physiologic parameters that are associated with higher risk for disease. Living in America doesn't have to be a recipe for a shorter, sicker life. In fact, with the proper knowledge about current health status combined with an action plan, anyone can beat the odds and increase their likelihood of a disease-free future.

We as a country cannot afford to be complacent about the devastating effects of chronic disease. Our healthcare costs are way out of line with the costs in other advanced countries. We spend more and get less for the dollars we spend. One of the goals of this guide is to provide practical information that will give every American a better chance to live as long as our friends across the ocean.

But remember, even though this book is full of actionable items, it's very important to develop a long-lasting dialogue with your healthcare provider. The future of healthcare will be driven by technological advances feeding data from mobile devices to the "cloud" for distribution and analysis. Healthcare providers will gradually learn to absorb vast amounts of data that will help them shape their medical interventions. This will evolve into a partnership between patients and medical professionals. Patients will be actively engaged in collecting data, instead of depending on office visits for data collection. For this new paradigm to work well, it is important for patients to have an accurate understanding of the basic principles of chronic disease prevention. The purpose of this guide is just that. Hopefully it will be a useful tool for patients as they become more active in the process of participating in a partnership with healthcare providers to lessen the burden of the chronic diseases that so often disrupt the last decades of life.

# What diseases am I most likely to die from?

The Centers for Disease Control and Prevention (CDC) are a great source of information about the diseases that are a threat to Americans. The following graphic shows the five major causes of death in 2014, and what percentage of each cause is deemed to be preventable.

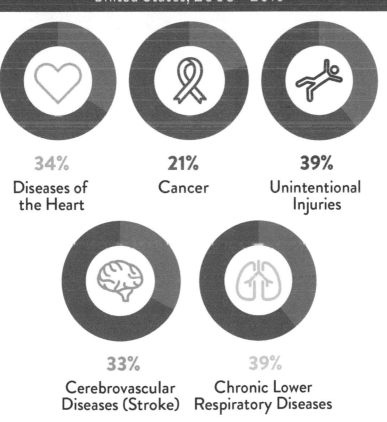

**Potentially Preventable Deaths from the Five Leading Causes of Death**

United States, 2008 - 2010

**34%**
Diseases of the Heart

**21%**
Cancer

**39%**
Unintentional Injuries

**33%**
Cerebrovascular Diseases (Stroke)

**39%**
Chronic Lower Respiratory Diseases

Together, these five categories account for 63% of all deaths. Because of successful medical and lifestyle interventions, such as medications for blood pressure control and cholesterol control, and the decrease in tobacco use, the mortality rate in 2014- 724.6 deaths per 100,000 population- was the lowest figure ever for Americans.

Since 1995, the number of Americans living with chronic disease has increased from 118 million to 171 million. This can be explained by a growing population over age 65 and by our successful treatment of cancer and cardiovascular disease, leaving more people alive for more years. With so many people living longer, and taking medications for multiple conditions, costs for healthcare continue to grow. Early awareness of the risk factors for future chronic disease, and a focused approach to lowering these risk factors, can have a major impact on delaying the onset of age-related disabilities.

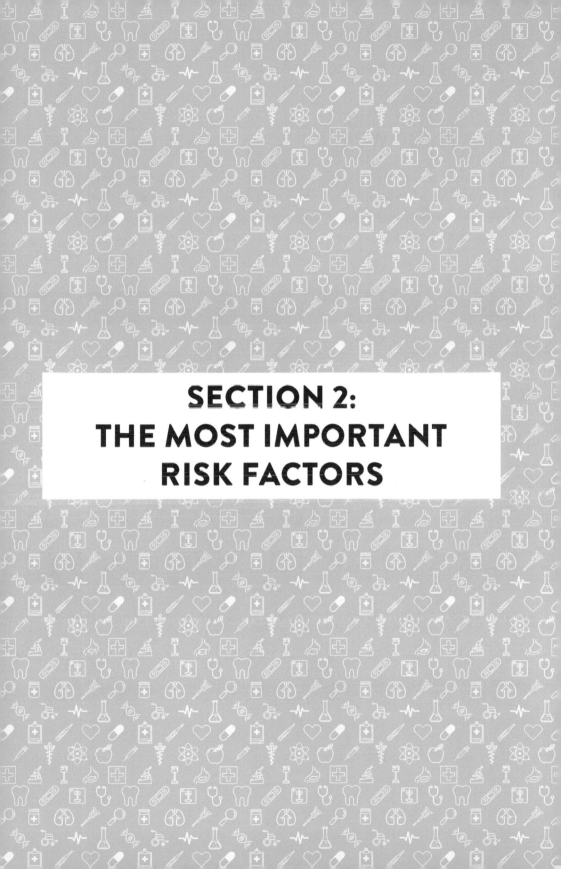

# SECTION 2:
# THE MOST IMPORTANT
# RISK FACTORS

# How is my weight?

At Scripps Executive Health, a large majority of our clients are overweight or obese. This is in keeping with a trend that has been going on for decades in America. The following graphic showing the growth of obesity illustrates how rapidly the waistlines of Americans have increased.

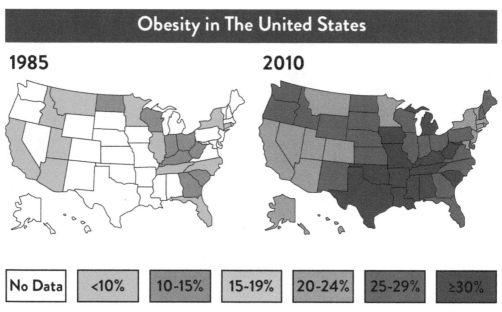

**Obesity in The United States**

1985

2010

| No Data | <10% | 10-15% | 15-19% | 20-24% | 25-29% | ≥30% |

www.cdc.gov/obesity/data

The most dramatic increases over the past half century have been in rates of obesity vs. rates of overweight. In the graph on the following page, you can see that from 1976 on the curve for obesity prevalence has angled upward in a truly frightening fashion.

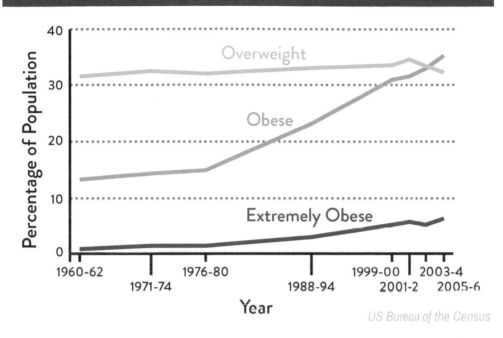

## Obesity in The United States

*US Bureau of the Census*

Being overweight or obese increases the risk for many chronic diseases. This makes it a very important metric for assessing how healthy you are. There are several ways to assess weight status. Body mass index is used to define overweight and obesity and is a ratio of weight to height.

## Calculate Your BMI

your weight (lbs):
$$\frac{\text{_____} \times 703}{\text{_____}^{2\ (squared)}} = $$ Your BMI
your height (in): _____

or

your weight (kg):
$$\frac{\text{_____}}{\text{_____}^{2\ (squared)}} = $$ Your BMI
your height (m): _____

Although BMI was originally conceived as a metric to study the relationship between weight and height during growth from birth to adulthood, after World War II it became the standard for quantifying excess weight. Weight adjusted for height is strongly correlated with body fat, but it is also correlated with body build- more muscular people will have higher BMIs. It also doesn't differentiate between subcutaneous fat and abdominal fat. Body mass index is a practical way to categorize people, but has significant limitations.

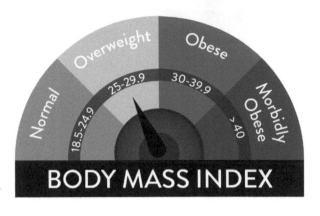

Another method to classify weight status is percent body fat-

## Ideal Body Fat Percentage Chart

| Description | Men | Women |
|---|---|---|
| Essential Fat | 2-5% | 10-13% |
| Athletes | 6-13% | 14-20% |
| Fitness | 14-17% | 21-24% |
| Average | 18-24% | 25-31% |
| Obese | 25%+ | 32%+ |

*American Council on Exercise*

The chart shows categories of weight based on percent body fat. Women have higher relative levels of fat compared to men so that they have adequate energy reserves during pregnancy. If a woman's percent body fat drops too low, she will stop ovulating.

Percent body fat is not as easy to measure as BMI or waist circumference, so we tend not to see it used as frequently. Body mass index is used universally to categorize weight status, and waist circumference is incorporated into the definition of metabolic syndrome (discussed later in the guide). But percent body fat is a very important indicator of health status.

The two main types of fat in the body are subcutaneous fat and visceral, or abdominal fat. The distinction is important, because they behave differently. Subcutaneous fat is not as dangerous as abdominal fat. Subcutaneous fat, in addition to providing an energy storage system, serves to cushion and insulate our bodies, and is more prominent in women. Abdominal fat is more metabolically active, and in the presence of excessive fat and/or excessive calories in the diet, releases large amounts of free fatty acids (storage fats can be in the form of free fatty acids or triglycerides. Triglycerides contain 3 fatty acid molecules attached to a short chain called glycerol). The free fatty acids travel directly to the liver through the portal vein.

The liver metabolizes the free fatty acids into triglycerides or glucose. If the liver is overwhelmed with free fatty acids, it begins to develop insulin resistance. As a result, it does not respond to insulin normally. Insulin signals the liver to stop making glucose. In insulin resistance, the liver continues to release glucose into the circulation, thus raising levels and triggering more insulin secretion. Over time, fat deposits build up in the liver and trigger chronic inflammation and fatty liver disease. Excess fatty acids also enter the general circulation and accumulate in other organs, including fat cells, muscle cells and the pancreas. This worsens insulin resistance and ultimately, can lead to diabetes.

Genes help determine where fat is deposited. Gender also plays a role, with women less likely before menopause to deposit fat in the abdominal cavity.

## Same Amount of Total Fat Mass
### Different Distribution of Fat

HEALTHIER    LESS HEALTHY

2x Visceral Fat

The graphic shows CT scans through the abdomen for 2 men. Both have the same amount of body fat (fat mass). But the person on the right has much more abdominal, or visceral fat.

Since few people undergo CT scans to measure their visceral fat, we use less sophisticated but still relatively powerful methods to capture this risk. Abdominal obesity increases risk for hypertension, abnormal blood lipids, diabetes, and coronary artery disease.

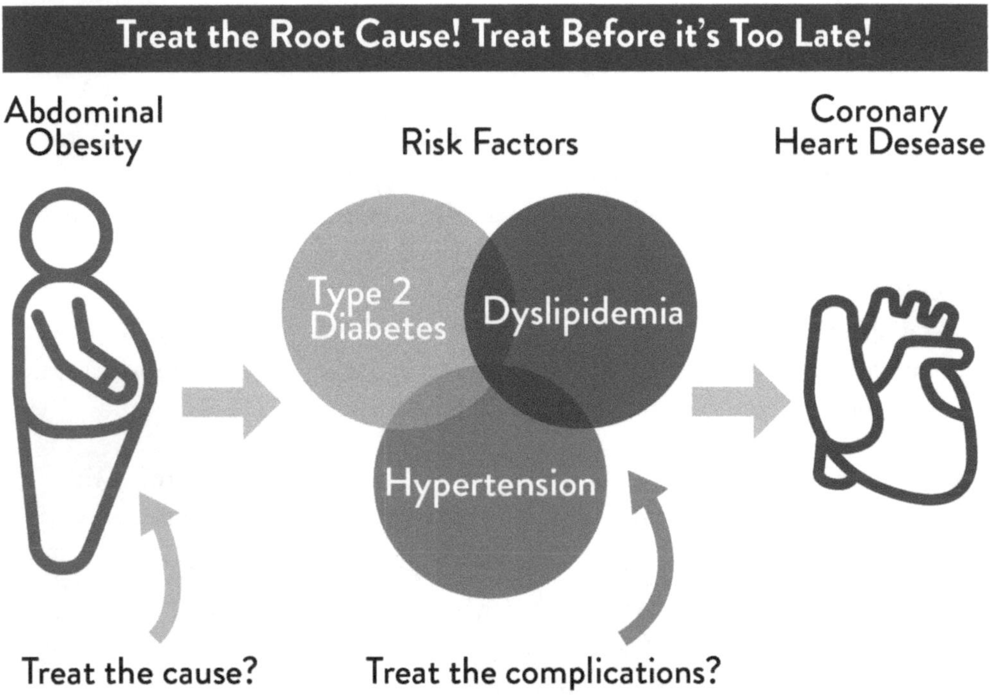

## Treat the Root Cause! Treat Before it's Too Late!

Abdominal
Obesity

Risk Factors

Coronary
Heart Desease

Type 2
Diabetes

Dyslipidemia

Hypertension

Treat the cause?

Treat the complications?

Two commonly used measurements are waist circumference and waist to hip ratio. Waist circumference is one of the five criteria used to diagnose metabolic syndrome, which we discuss later in the guide.

Waist to hip ratio has been shown in well-designed studies to be a better predictor of heart disease than BMI.

| | | Small Waist | Large Waist | Very Large Waist |
|---|---|---|---|---|
| | Women: | < 31.5 in | 31.5 - 35.5 in | > 35.5 in |
| | Men: | < 37 in | 37- 40 in | > 40 in |
| **Body Mass Index** | Overweight BMI: 25-29.99 | No Increased Risk | Increased Risk | High Risk |
| | Obese BMI: 30-34.99 | Increased Risk | High Risk | Very High Risk |

At the Center for Executive Health, we calculate BMI, waist circumference, waist to hip ratio and percent body fat.

# How is my blood pressure?

High blood pressure, or hypertension, is the most common cardiovascular disease. Its prevalence goes up with age-

- 50% of Americans over age 50
- 75% over age 75
- 90% over age 90

Although there are many risk factors, here are a few key ones-

- Family history
- Sedentary lifestyle
- Obesity
- High sodium, low potassium diets

- Chronic high stress levels
- Sleep apnea
- Certain hormonal problems
- Excessive alcohol consumption

## Complications of High Blood Pressure

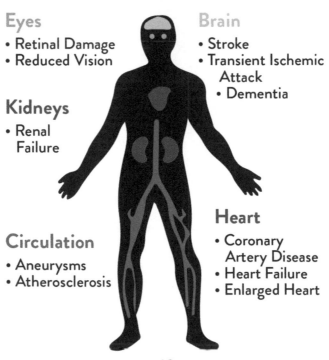

Eyes
- Retinal Damage
- Reduced Vision

Brain
- Stroke
- Transient Ischemic Attack
- Dementia

Kidneys
- Renal Failure

Circulation
- Aneurysms
- Atherosclerosis

Heart
- Coronary Artery Disease
- Heart Failure
- Enlarged Heart

Hypertension may develop silently, or, if the blood pressure is seriously elevated, may result in symptoms such as a headache, chest pain, shortness of breath or palpitations. Many of our clients are surprised when we find their blood pressure elevated. High blood pressure over many years causes damage to multiple organs, and the amount of damage is proportional to the length of time of the exposure to high blood pressure.

For this reason, early identification and treatment is very important.

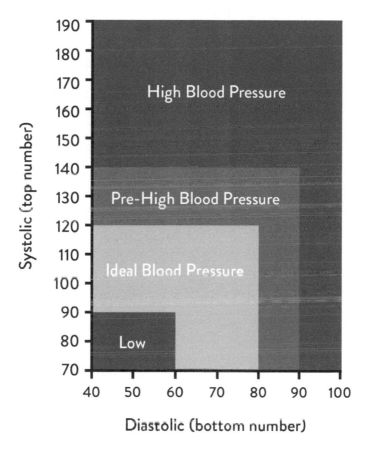

About 1 in 3 people will have high blood pressure in the doctor's office, but normal blood pressure at home. This is often referred to as white coat hypertension. It seems the act of having a medical professional take the blood pressure is stressful enough to cause a significant rise in blood pressure for a subset of people. Blood pressure readings at home are a more accurate indicator of risk. It is best to take two readings after resting quietly for a few minutes, and average the results. Do this on several occasions over the course of a week, perhaps 5-10 readings in all. Then average the systolic and diastolic readings. If the average systolic pressure is over 130 and or the average diastolic reading is over 85, then you may be a candidate for a blood pressure reduction program.

At Scripps, we perform a more advanced type of blood pressure measurement in addition to the standard brachial blood pressure (the brachial artery is accessed with the cuff just above the elbow). We use a device, called SphygmoCor, that can measure the blood pressure in the aorta using special sensors. As the left ventricle squeezes, the pressure in the aorta rises, peaks,

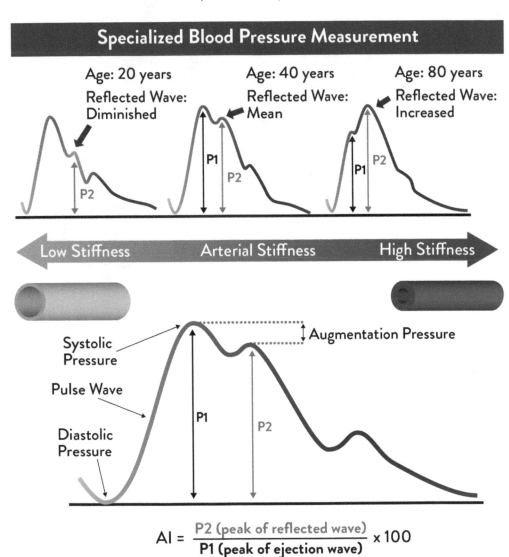

## Specialized Blood Pressure Measurement

Age: 20 years
Reflected Wave: Diminished

Age: 40 years
Reflected Wave: Mean

Age: 80 years
Reflected Wave: Increased

P1
P2

P1
P2

P1
P2

Low Stiffness     Arterial Stiffness     High Stiffness

Systolic Pressure

Pulse Wave

Diastolic Pressure

Augmentation Pressure

P1
P2

$$AI = \frac{P2 \text{ (peak of reflected wave)}}{P1 \text{ (peak of ejection wave)}} \times 100$$

and falls. In the diagram below, this a the P1 wave. The machine also can characterize the wave of blood that gets reflected back towards the heart when the aorta bifurcates in the pelvic region. This is called the P2 wave. The speed at which the reflected wave travels is proportional to arterial stiffness.

As can be seen in the diagram on the previous page, the reflected wave actually moves up the downward slope of the original wave. The reflected wave height, P2, divided by the original wave height, P1, times 100 equals the augmentation index, AI. In a young, elastic artery, the wave is smaller and occurs towards the end of the downward slope, giving a lower AI value. In a stiffer older artery, the wave moves back so fast that it occurs early after the peak of the forward wave, giving a higher AI. The SphygmoCor report actually calculates a vascular age based on arterial stiffness, which is proportional to the augmentation index. Generally, people who exercise regularly (particularly cardio exercise) have a vascular age significantly lower than their chronologic age.

High blood pressure can be lowered through lifestyle changes. The diagram below shows the range of benefit in blood pressure lowering for various lifestyle interventions. For those who are overweight or obese, losing weight can have a very significant effect on blood pressure. The DASH eating pattern is based on the DASH Diet, developed at NIH. It is high in fruits, vegetables and low fat sources of protein.

The first step in the development of hypertension is a condition called endothelial dysfunction. The endothelium is the innermost lining of the artery wall. When functioning normally, it secretes optimal amounts of nitric oxide, the powerful little molecule that relaxes the smooth muscle in the artery wall, and dilates the artery. Poor diet, lack of exercise and obesity can cause endothelial dysfunction, measured by a decrease in nitric oxide. This makes the artery more susceptible to both hypertension and atherosclerosis.

Loss of nitric oxide translates into an artery that is less capable of dilating. Medium-sized arteries throughout the body are constantly constricting and dilating to direct blood flow to the organs that are most active at any given moment. In hypertension, the smooth muscles are unable to dilate normally. As a result, the heart has to beat more forcefully to overcome the resistance to flow caused by the abnormally constricted arteries.

Over many years, the arteries become less and less able to dilate normally.

In the initial years of hypertension, lifestyle changes my be all that is needed to restore normal levels of nitric oxide and normal endothelial function. But eventually medications become necessary to bring blood pressure back down to a normal level.

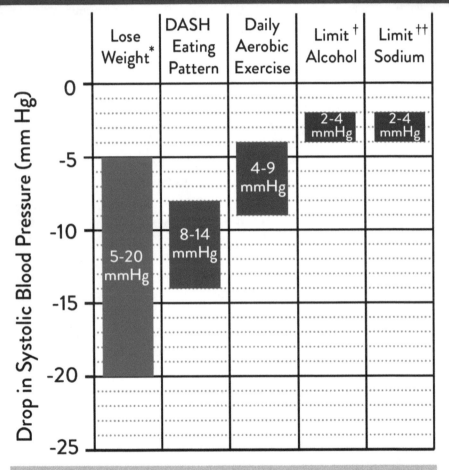

## Approximate Reduction in Systolic Blood Pressure With Diet and Lifestyle Changes

| | Lose Weight* | DASH Eating Pattern | Daily Aerobic Exercise | Limit † Alcohol | Limit †† Sodium |
|---|---|---|---|---|---|
| | 5-20 mmHg | 8-14 mmHg | 4-9 mmHg | 2-4 mmHg | 2-4 mmHg |

*Drop in Systolic Blood Pressure (mm Hg)* — vertical axis scale: 0, -5, -10, -15, -20, -25

* 22 lb weight loss in overweight/obese adults
** Dietary Approaches to Stop Hypertension
† Maximum 1 drink/day for Women, 2/day for Men
†† Sodium Reduced by ~ 1,200 mg/day

# What supplements may lower blood pressure?

Certain supplements have been shown to have a beneficial effect on endothelial function. In the setting of a healthy diet high in fruits, vegetables, whole grains, seafood, nuts and healthy oils, their effects would most likely not be great. But if diet quality is not optimal, they will have a more pronounced beneficial effect. Here is a list of those supplements that have been shown to potentially improve endothelial function and lower blood pressure-

- Coenzyme Q10
- Omega-3 fish oil
- Garlic extract
- Potassium and magnesium
- Alpha lipoic acid
- Melatonin at night
- Vitamin C
- Zinc

# What are the safest medications for high blood pressure?

If your blood pressure is consistently over 140/90, there is less chance that you will be able to lower it quickly through lifestyle changes or with supplements. It is always possible that as you lose weight or improve your diet, you may be able to transition to lower doses of blood pressure medications, a lower number of medications, or even stop altogether. But it is dangerous to postpone taking blood pressure medications, as end organ damage is proportional to the length of time the blood pressure is high, and the severity of the hypertension. As hypertension becomes more advanced, it becomes harder to reverse the changes in the artery wall, and more aggressive treatment regimens, with multiple medications, may be necessary.

The safest blood pressure medications are those with the fewest side effects. Below is a list of blood pressure medications by order of safest to least safe-

- Angiotensin receptor blockers (ARBs)
- Ace inhibitors
- Calcium channel blockers
- Low dose thiazide diuretics

- Low dose beta blockers
- Spironolactone
- Clonidine
- Hydralazine

In general, the lower the dose, the safer the medication. Higher doses of beta blockers can cause dangerously slow heart rates in some people. Higher doses of diuretics can produce electrolyte abnormalities such as low serum potassium levels. In people with kidney disease, spironolactone can cause high serum potassium levels. It is often preferable to take lower doses of two or three blood pressure medications versus a high dose of one.

# What are the blood lipids?

In the popular mind, cholesterol is considered a dangerous substance that blocks arteries and causes heart attacks and strokes. But cholesterol in reality is a very important molecule found in every cell membrane and is a building block for many hormones, including cortisol, aldosterone, testosterone, progesterone and estrogen, as well as vitamin D. It also is used to produce bile acids, the molecules that help with digestion of fats in the intestine.

Cholesterol was labeled public enemy number one in the war against heart disease in the 1960s. Back then, blood tests were quite primitive. It was found that people with very high levels of cholesterol in their blood had a very high risk for heart attacks. Also, based on a flawed study called the Seven Countries Study, cholesterol and saturated fat in the diet were implicated as the main drivers of high cholesterol in the blood. Over the past few decades, our understanding of lipid (fat) metabolism has vastly improved. We now know that the cholesterol in the blood is made in the liver and is inserted into little spherical particles that contain mainly triglycerides. So, cholesterol levels in the blood go up when the liver makes more triglycerides. The liver can make triglycerides from glucose, a sugar, or from fatty acids. So when the diet has excessive amounts of fats or sugars, the liver makes large amounts of these particles, called very low density lipoprotein (VLDL) particles. VLDL particles have a ratio of triglyceride to cholesterol of about 5 to 1, but this ratio goes up when triglyceride production goes up.

Once these VLDL particles are released from the liver into the circulation, they unload their triglyceride cargo into either fat or muscle cells. After triglyceride removal, the VLDL particle first turns into an IDL (intermediate density lipoprotein) particle and then turns into an LDL (low density lipoprotein) particle. VLDL, IDL and LDL particles can enter the artery wall and initiate the process called atherosclerosis.

The third blood lipid particle is the high density lipoprotein (HDL) particle. This contains cholesterol for transport back to the liver. Studies have shown that higher levels of the HDL particle are protective, thus the cholesterol in the

25

HDL particle is sometimes called good cholesterol while the cholesterol in the LDL particle is called bad cholesterol. It's really all the same cholesterol, just being carried in different particles!

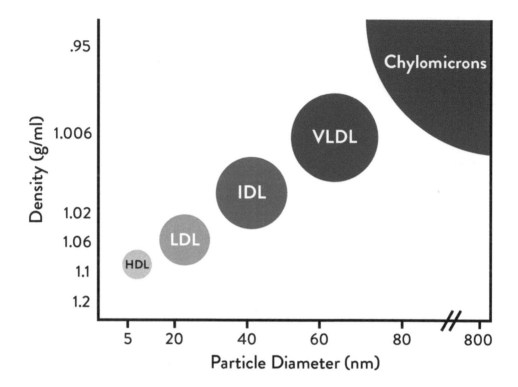

As the diagram above shows, there are five kinds of lipoprotein particles that carry cholesterol and triglycerides. The chylomicron particle is produced in the small intestine and carries triglycerides and cholesterol from the food we eat to the liver. Its large size prevents it from entering the artery wall and causing damage. The intermediate density lipoprotein (IDL) particle is an intermediate stage in the conversion of VLDL to LDL. All of these particles together comprise the blood lipids.

# How is my lipid panel?

Cholesterol levels are reported on the lipid panel, along with triglyceride levels. There are three categories of cholesterol: total cholesterol, LDL cholesterol and HDL cholesterol. Since total cholesterol is the sum of all the cholesterol in the lipoprotein particles, it includes cholesterol in the potentially harmful particles (LDL, VLDL and IDL) and in the protective HDL particle. This means that when someone has a large amount of HDL cholesterol it will raise the total cholesterol to a level that might appear too high. Total cholesterol is not a veryuseful metric for risk, unless it is very high or very low.

LDL cholesterol and triglycerides are both associated with a higher risk for cardiovascular disease. Triglycerides are also associated with higher risk for diabetes. An optimal LDL cholesterol for someone with no history of cardiovascular disease is less than 100 mg/dL. For those with a history of heart attack or stroke, a safer level is below 70 mg/dL. As LDL cholesterol rises, so does risk for heart attacks and strokes. LDL cholesterol is not significantly affected by a recent meal, so it is no longer considered necessary to fast before having it checked. HDL cholesterol also can be checked in a fasting or non-fasting state. Less than 40mg/dL is associated with higher risk. Over 60mg/dL is associated with lower risk, and is therefore optimal. Triglycerides rise quickly after ingesting food, particularly high fat foods, and can take several hours to return to fasting levels. A fasting triglyceride level of less than 100 is optimal. A non-fasting lipid panel is better than a fasting lipid panel at detecting problems with triglycerides. This is because studies have shown that the post-prandial (post-meal) triglyceride level is a better predictor of risk than the fasting triglyceride level.

Going back to the lipoprotein particles, triglycerides are primarily carried in chylomicrons, VLDL and IDL particles. Chylomicrons, as mentioned above, cannot enter the artery wall, but VLDL and IDL particles can, and therefore are associated with risk for the development of atherosclerosis.

Knowing your lipoprotein particle numbers is a more accurate way to evaluate risk when compared to the lipid panel. Let's compare the two:

| LIPID PANEL | LIPOPROTEIN PARTICLE |
|---|---|
| LDL cholesterol | LDL particle |
| HDL cholesterol | HDL particle |
| Triglycerides | VLDL, IDL particle |

LDL, VLDL and IDL particles can all enter the artery wall and initiate atherosclerosis. LDL cholesterol level will underestimate risk when triglycerides are high. A good way to assess risk in the setting of high triglycerides is to calculate non-HDL cholesterol. This is done by subtracting HDL cholesterol from total cholesterol. This tells you the total amount of cholesterol in the dangerous particles (LDL, VLDL and IDL). The optimal non-HDL cholesterol is 30 mg/dL higher than the corresponding optimal LDL cholesterol.

# How does cholesterol damage my arteries?

Now that you know about the lipoprotein particles, you know that it is more accurate to say "how are the lipoprotein particles damaging my arteries?" The dangerous lipoprotein particles can passively diffuse across the artery lining (the endothelium). The more particles there are, the more will diffuse into the artery. Also, when triglycerides are high, the LDL particles end up losing some of their cholesterol in exchange for triglycerides. This tends to convert the LDL particles into a small and dense form, and makes them more prone to oxidation. The oxidized lipoprotein particles in the wall can trigger an inflammatory response. You body sees them as dangerous and sends in white blood cells to remove them. Unfortunately, this triggers an inflammatory response that drives the production of the plaque that is responsible for heart attacks, strokes and other vascular problems.

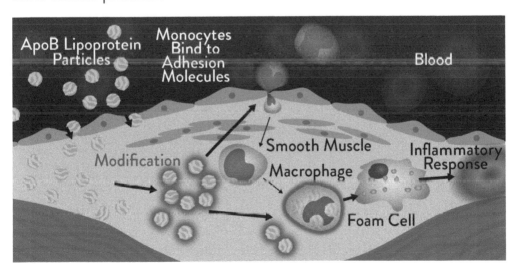

In the drawing above, the ApoB lipoprotein particles are the dangerous LDL, VLDL and IDL particles. The modification is oxidation and/or glycation (glucose attaching to the particle). Both of these modifications can trigger the monocytes to enter the wall. The monocytes are converted to macrophages that engulf the particles. This results in the formation of a foam cell, a cell filled with the modified cholesterol-carrying particles. When this process occurs chronically, it leads to plaque formation. A plaque with a high number of macrophages and foam cells is called an unstable plaque, because it has a tendency to rupture through the artery wall. When this happens, a clot forms at the rupture point. The clot could obstruct the artery and cause a heart attack (in the coronaries) or part of it could break loose and be carried downstream (in the arteries going to the brain), causing a stroke.

# How do I know if my artery wall has plaque?

There are two tests used to screen for plaque build-up in the arteries. Unfortunately, because these are screening tests, they are usually not covered by your insurance. The best test for determining your risk for a heart attack is called a coronary artery calcium score. It is done by taking a low radiation dose CT scan of the heart. Each of the 40 or so slices through the heart contains segments of the three coronary arteries. A normal artery appears grey. If the artery has more than just a tiny amount of plaque, the plaque will have some calcium in it, which appears white on the scan slice. Special software is used to quantify the amount of calcium in each visible plaque. All the plaque scores are added up to produce the coronary artery calcium score.

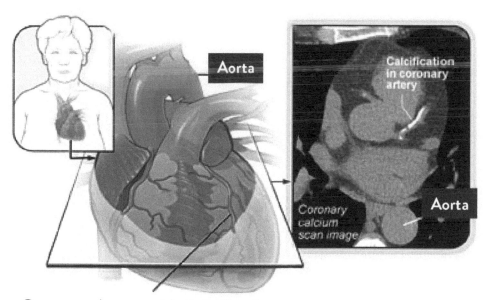

**Coronary Artery with Calcification**

*NIH National Heart, Blood & Lung Institute*

The higher the coronary artery calcium score, the higher the risk for a heart attack. In addition to the absolute score, the test provides a percentile score. This compares the person to an age-gender matched group. A person with a score that is higher than 75% of the age-gender matched group would have a percentile score of 75%. This is useful for predicting future risk. A 50 year old might have a mild category calcium score, but be in the 80th percentile. This means that the person's future risk for a heart attack is in the top 20%. By finding this out at age 50, lifestyle changes and possibly medications can be instituted to lower future risk.

## Calcium Score Guidelines

| Total Score | Plaque Burden | Risk Category |
|---|---|---|
| 0 | None | Very Low |
| 1-10 | Minimal | Low |
| 11-100 | Mild | Moderate |
| 101-400 | Moderate | Moderate High |
| Over 400 | Extensive | High |

The other test for identifying potentially harmful plaque or cholesterol in the artery wall is an ultrasound of the carotid arteries. The left and right carotid arteries are on either side of the neck, and bring blood to the brain. They are easily accessible with ultrasound (unlike the coronaries, which are too small and too far below the body surface to be examined with ultrasound).

The ultrasound images obtained will reveal whether the artery wall contains plaque, and if so, one can categorize the plaque as minimal, mild, moderate or severe. The greater the amount of plaque volume, the greater the risk for stroke or heart attack. Carotid plaque is directly related to stroke risk, since the clot produced by a ruptured plaque will travel up to the brain. But the presence of excessive plaque in carotids suggests the possibility of excessive plaque in the coronaries as well. Therefore, this test can predict both stroke and heart attack risk.

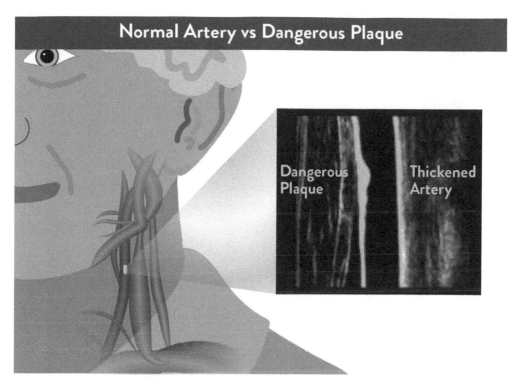

The carotid ultrasound can also be used to measure the thickness of the carotid artery wall. This is called intimal medial thickness, or IMT. Measurements are taken in thousands of a millimeter. Databases permit the comparison of a measurement to a large population. Measurement results are reported by quartile. The lowest risk quartile means a result in the lowest 25% of the population, age-gender matched. The highest risk quartile is above the 75th percentile. The thicker the wall, the more cholesterol it contains. In general, cholesterol accumulates as we age, so the IMT goes up with age. Treatments or lifestyle changes aimed at lowering LDL cholesterol or raising HDL cholesterol can result in gradual thinning of the wall as cholesterol is removed. The IMT has also been shown to be related to stroke and heart attack risk, but is not as predictive as the presence of plaque.

# Should I be taking a statin?

Statins are medications that lower LDL cholesterol and LDL particles. They also have anti-inflammatory and anti-platelet (platelets are the little cells that initiate clot formation) properties. They are among the most studied medications in the world. Many people refuse to take them because of their perceived risks. Unfortunately, this means many people are subjecting themselves to a higher risk for heart attacks and strokes.

Multiple lines of research have proven beyond a doubt that as LDL cholesterol goes up, risk for cardiovascular disease goes up. Nonetheless, a decision to take a statin should not be based solely on LDL cholesterol level. Very high levels of LDL cholesterol (greater than 190mg/dL) warrant taking a statin regardless of whether other risk factors are present. But only a small percentage of people have such high LDL cholesterol. Since most people have LDL cholesterol levels less than 150, other risk factors are more important than the LDL cholesterol level.

Anyone who has had a heart attack or stroke (unless the stroke was related to atrial fibrillation) should be taking a statin. This population of people has a high risk for another heart attack or stroke. Taking a statin will reduce that risk by an amount proportional to the LDL lowering. If the LDL cholesterol is lowered by 50%, risk will go down by about 40-50%, compared to someone not taking a statin.

The 40-50% risk reduction is in relative risk not absolute risk. What is the difference between the two? If your risk of a heart attack before taking the statin was 20% and your risk after taking the statin is 10%, this represents a 50% relative risk reduction and a 10% absolute risk reduction (your risk has been halved by the statin, but in absolute terms, it has gone down 10%). This brings up a very important concept, called "number needed to treat" or NNT.

NNT is the number needed to treat for any particular absolute risk reduction. If the absolute risk reduction is 10%, then to prevent 1 heart attack you need to treat 10 people. To prevent 100 heart attacks, you need to treat 1000 people.

If you have a 50% risk of a heart attack in the next 10 years, and a particular dose of a statin lowers relative risk by 50%, your risk after taking the statin goes down to 25%. This also is a 25% absolute risk reduction. At this high risk level, only 4 people have to be treated to prevent 1 person from having a heart

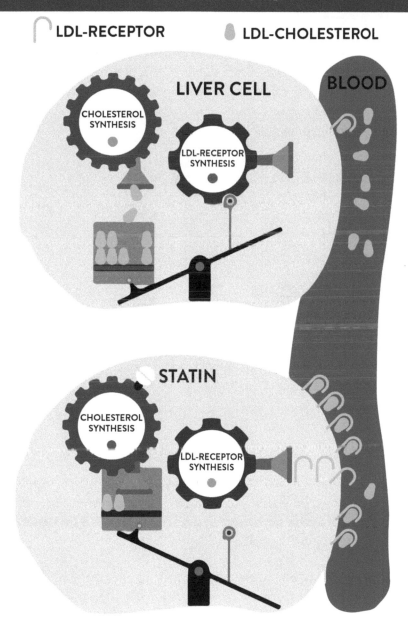

attack (NNT is the inverse of the absolute risk reduction, or 1/ARR where ARR is absolute risk reduction- so in this case NNT is 1/0.25=4).

Now let's consider the case where your risk of having a heart attack is 2% over the next 10 years. If your statin therapy lowers relative risk by 50%, your risk goes down to 1% over 10 years. However, your absolute risk reduction is only 1%. This means NNT is 100/0.1= 1000. In this scenario, 1000 people have to be treated to prevent 1 heart attack.

Now you can understand why it is so important to know your absolute risk of having a heart attack or stroke before deciding whether or not to take a statin. Cardiovascular risk can be calculated by adding up your number of risk factors. Many such calculators can be found on the web. But you can get a rough idea of your risk by simply adding up your risk factors. Here is a list of risk factors:

- Age over 45 for men and 55 for women
- HDL cholesterol less than 40 for men and 50 for women
- Diabetes or pre-diabetes
- High blood pressure
- Cigarette smoking
- Obesity
- Sedentary lifestyle
- LDL cholesterol over 160-190
- Chronically high stress levels
- Family history of premature cardiovascular disease (first degree relative with onset of disease before age 60)
- Triglyceride level higher than 150-200
- C-reactive protein (CRP) higher than 3
- Metabolic syndrome
- Sleeping less than 7-8 hours per night
- Sleep apnea

The greater the number of risk factors you have, the higher your risk. Another powerful way to assess your risk is to obtain a coronary artery calcium score or a carotid ultrasound assessment of plaque and wall thickness (see section "How do I know if my artery wall has plaque?).

Statins prevent adverse cardiovascular events. There are two kinds of prevention- primary and secondary. Secondary prevention means preventing another adverse event in someone who has already had one. Absolute risk reduction is generally higher in this population because absolute risk is higher. But consider the fact that when a heart attack occurs, many people die immediately, because the sudden cessation of blood flow to the heart muscle triggers a lethal arrhythmia, called ventricular fibrillation. This means many people don't get a chance for secondary prevention. Also, heart attacks can irreversibly destroy heart muscle and strokes can lead to permanent disability. So, is it really prudent to refrain from taking a statin until after you have had a potentially devastating adverse cardiovascular event?

Primary prevention means preventing your first adverse cardiovascular event. If successful, then the heart remains intact and the brain remains intact. This is very desirable. Primary prevention means reducing your risk profile, as defined by the risk factors listed above. Many of these risk factors can be successfully lowered by improving your lifestyle. So statin therapy is only one method for lowering risk. Any lifestyle change that removes items from the list above can potentially be just as effective as statin therapy, if the changes are long term.

# Should I be taking aspirin?

Many of the considerations listed above for statin therapy apply to aspirin therapy. In secondary prevention, aspirin is a powerful tool for reducing risk. In primary prevention, its use should be restricted to those who have a moderate to high risk for adverse cardiovascular events. In absolute terms, this means a greater than 10% 10-year risk. The US Preventive Services Task Force actually refines this further by recommending use to those with intermediate to higher risk who are 50-69 years of age, and who are not at increased risk for bleeding. Their analysis finds insufficient evidence to support its use in those under age 50 and over age 70. The Task Force also recommends it for use in the same population for prevention of colon cancer.

Anti-Clot                                    Anti-Inflammation

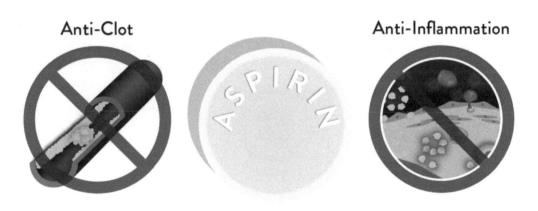

# How is my level of fitness?

At the Scripps Center for Executive health, a treadmill test is an important component of the comprehensive examination. Cardiologists routinely perform treadmill tests in patients who have chest pain to rule out heart disease. In that setting, the treadmill test is called a stress test. However, the treadmill test also serves another very important function. It can measure fitness level as a function of time endurance on a treadmill. A standardized protocol is utilized that takes the client through increasing stages of difficulty, as the

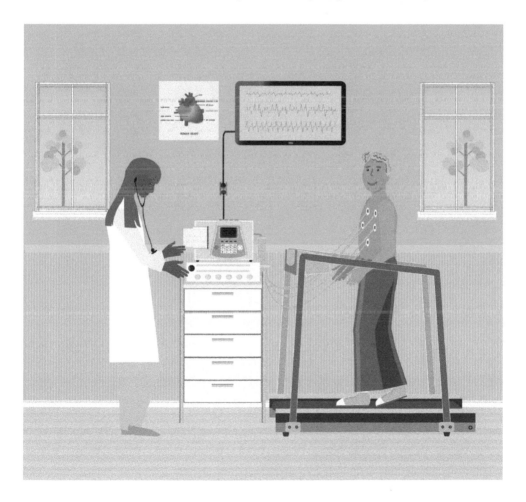

speed and incline of the treadmill are increased every 3 minutes. The average person in middle age becomes too fatigued to continue at about 9-10 minutes of exercise, either at the end of stage 3 or the beginning of stage 4. More fit individuals can continue to exercise into stage 5, stage 6 or higher. During the treadmill, the clients must not hold onto the bar at the front of the treadmill. Holding the bar, while important in older patients being tested for heart disease to maintain balance, is a form of cheating when measuring fitness.

The seminal study reporting the relationship between how long one can exercise on a treadmill and how long one will live was done at the Cooper Clinic in Dallas. It appeared in the Journal of the American Medical Association on November 3, 1989. It was entitled "Physical Fitness and All-Cause Mortality-A Prospective Study of Healthy Men and Women." More than 13,000 men and women who had performed treadmill fitness tests were followed for an average of 8 years. Here is a quote from the article:

> "There were 240 deaths in men and 43 deaths in women. Age-adjusted all-cause mortality rates declined across physical fitness quintiles from 64.0 per 10 000 person-years in the least-fit men to 18.6 per 10 000 person-years in the most-fit men. Corresponding values for women were 39.5 per 10 000 person-years to 8.5 per 10 000 person-years. These trends remained after statistical adjustment for age, smoking habit, cholesterol level, systolic blood pressure, fasting blood glucose level, parental history of coronary heart disease, and follow-up interval. Lower mortality rates in higher fitness categories also were seen for cardiovascular disease and cancer of combined sites. Attributable risk estimates for all-cause mortality indicated that low physical fitness was an important risk factor in both men and women. Higher levels of physical fitness appear to delay all-cause mortality primarily due to lowered rates of cardiovascular disease and cancer."

This remarkable benefit from being fit translates into a 70% reduction in mortality rates for men and an 80% reduction for women! Numerous other studies have shown the beneficial effects of exercise. There is no simple answer to why an active lifestyle confers such a strong survival advantage. But we can begin by acknowledging that a sedentary lifestyle, with its attendant risks for the accumulation of dangerous levels of fat deposits throughout the body, and its adverse effects on muscle, bone and heart strength, causes a general deterioration of functional status that increases the likelihood of premature disease and death. An active lifestyle has beneficial effects on the immune system, energy balance, brain function, mental well being, sleep quality, cardiac function, pulmonary function and stress hormone status.

In the language of Darwin, survival of the fittest refers to those members of a species best able to survive in a potentially hostile environment, thereby assuring that their genes become more prevalent in future generations through natural selection. But survival of the fittest could also refer to the survival advantage noted above. A regular exercise program and an active lifestyle increase fitness, and those who are most fit survive longest.

There are several elements of the Scripps Executive Exam that correlate with fitness:

- Body mass index (BMI)- fit people are more likely to have a BMI less than 25, although this is less likely to apply to body builders and those with naturally more muscle and bone mass (endomorphs).
- Waist circumference- a measure of abdominal cavity fat, inversely correlated with fitness.
- Waist to hip ratio- also negatively correlated with fitness.
- Percent body fat- inversely correlated with fitness. However, chronic disease or malnutrition are other causes of decreased percent body fat.
- Metabolic syndrome- the more criteria you meet, the less fit you are.
- Arterial wall stiffness- as measured with the core blood pressure. Lower vascular age directly correlates with fitness.
- Resting heart rate- lower heart rates are associated with fitness, although medications and cardiac conditions can also lower heart rate.
- Treadmill test using the Bruce Protocol- achieving 11 minutes or higher without holding the bar is associated with superior fitness (completing most of stage 4 or higher).
- HDL-cholesterol level- directly correlated with fitness.
- Triglyceride level- fitness associated with lower triglyceride levels.
- Hemoglobin A1c- fitness associated with lower risk for prediabetes or diabetes

# Do I have metabolic syndrome?

A sedentary lifestyle and/or a diet with excessive fats and sugars creates the perfect environment for metabolic syndrome. As the term suggests, metabolic syndrome is a condition characterized by disrupted energy metabolism. The initial step is the accumulation of fat in the abdominal cavity (abdominal or visceral fat). The excessive amounts of fat lead to an elevation of triglycerides in the blood and in other organs, such as the liver. This in turn leads to a lower HLD cholesterol level as triglycerides replace cholesterol in the HDL particle. The excessive amounts of triglycerides can also produce a condition called insulin resistance. This means that certain organs and tissues throughout the body do not respond normally to insulin signaling. Insulin signals open up channels that allow the entry of sugar (glucose) molecules into the cells. Since the glucose cannot enter the cells, blood glucose levels stay elevated after a meal. This signals the pancreas to keep releasing more insulin into the blood stream. As a result, both blood glucose and blood insulin levels are high. High

## Metabolic Syndrome

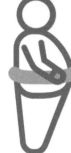

**Waist Circumference**
greater than
40" in men
35" in women

**Blood Pressure**
greater than
130/85 mmHg

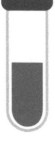

**Triglyceride Level**
greater than
150mg/dL

**HDL Cholesterol**
less than
40 mg/dL in men
50 mg/dL in women

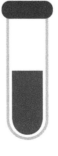

**Fasting Glucose Level**
greater than
100 mg/dL

insulin levels tend to raise blood pressure. So metabolic syndrome has 5 criteria, and having 3 or more of the criteria defines having the condition:

- Waist circumference greater than 40" in men or 35" in women
- Triglyceride level greater than 150
- HDL cholesterol less than 40 in men or 50 in women
- Fasting glucose level greater than 100
- Blood pressure greater than 130/85

Having metabolic syndrome creates the perfect environment for many diseases:

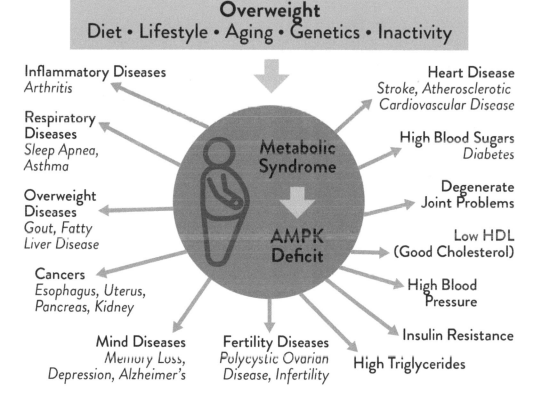

Why would metabolic syndrome have so many dangerous consequences? For the simple reason that evolutionary success depended upon careful energy utilization. Our bodies are designed to adjust metabolic processes based on the amount of energy available to our cells. When energy levels are high, cells work on anabolic processes (building molecules such as proteins, triglycerides and glycogen). When energy levels are low, cells switch towards catabolic energy processes (breaking down sugar and fat molecules for energy production).

In conditions of chronic high fat/sugar intake and low physical activity the mechanisms that control energy balance are disrupted, because during our evolution survival depended upon storing energy and using it sparingly. Survival never depended upon disposing of excess calories. Therefore we did not evolve metabolic pathways for this purpose . When we eat too much, we store more and more fat. Fat cells have limits to how much fat they can hold. When these limits are reached, the fat cells are stressed, triggering an inflammatory response. This leads to chronic low grade inflammation, a risk factor for cardiovascular disease and cancer. Excess fat also builds up in the liver, causing liver inflammation and chronic fatty liver disease. Excess fat also ends up in lots of other places, playing havoc on normal metabolic processes.

There is a very important molecule in all our cells called AMPK. This molecule can sense the amount of energy available to the cell. If energy levels are high, AMPK activity is suppressed. If energy levels are low, AMPK is activated. Activated AMPK directs the mitochondria to burn fat and glucose to make more energy (in the form of ATP). Healthy levels of activated AMPK are associated with insulin sensitivity and longevity. Suppressed levels of AMPK are associated with insulin resistance, diabetes and high risk for the chronic diseases of aging.

# What is my risk for diabetes?

Diabetes develops slowly over many years. There are several ways to assess your risk for this condition. Earlier in the book we discussed metabolic syndrome. If you have metabolic syndrome, your risk for diabetes is high. Recall that the metabolic syndrome criteria included waist circumference (a measure of obesity), and triglyceride level. Obesity can lead to high blood triglyceride levels. Abnormally high levels of triglycerides inside cells can disrupt insulin signaling and cause insulin resistance. Insulin resistance is essentially pre-diabetes.

## Prediabetes
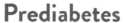

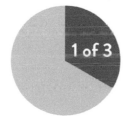
**86 Million**
American adults
have prediabetes

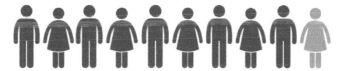

But only **1 of 10** know they have prediabetes

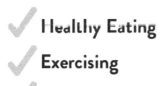 Healthy Eating

Exercising

Losing Weight

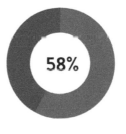
**58%**

Reduce your risk of develping type 2 diabetes by 58%

Changing your lifestyle proved **more** effective than medication in preventing onset of type 2 diabetes.

A very important test that we perform at Scripps as part of the executive health exam is called the hemoglobin A1c test. This measures how much glucose has become attached to the hemoglobin in the red blood cells. Since hemoglobin lasts for about 3 months before being recycled, the % of hemoglobin with glucose attached is a rough estimate of the average blood sugar over the last 3 months.

Less than 5.7% A1c is normal, 5.7% to 6.5% is an indicator of pre-diabetes, and over 6.5% suggests diabetes is present. The following table shows the equivalent average 3 month blood sugar levels for a range of A1c values. Once a person has diabetes, the A1c is used to track the response to therapeutic interventions, consisting of lifestyle changes and medications.

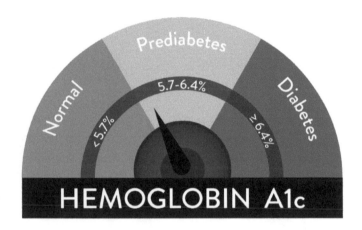

| A1c% | 3 Month Average Blood Sugar |
|------|------|
| 4.0 | 65 |
| 4.5 | 83 |
| 5.0 | 100 |
| 5.5 | 118 |
| 6.0 | 135 |
| 6.5 | 153 |
| 7.0 | 170 |
| 7.5 | 187 |
| 8.0 | 204 |
| 8.5 | 222 |
| 9.0 | 240 |
| 9.5 | 258 |
| 10.0 | 275 |
| 10.5 | 293 |
| 11.0 | 310 |
| 11.5 | 328 |
| 12.0 | 345 |

Typically, the goal for a diabetic is to keep their A1c below 6.5-7%.

Because of the obesity epidemic, the risk for diabetes is increasing at a rapid pace. The set of maps on the following page compare the increase in obesity in America with the increase in diabetes.

*Diabetes Care, Volume 25, Number 2, February 2002*

# Age-Adjusted Prevalence of Obesity and Diagnosed Diabetes Among US Adults

## Obesity

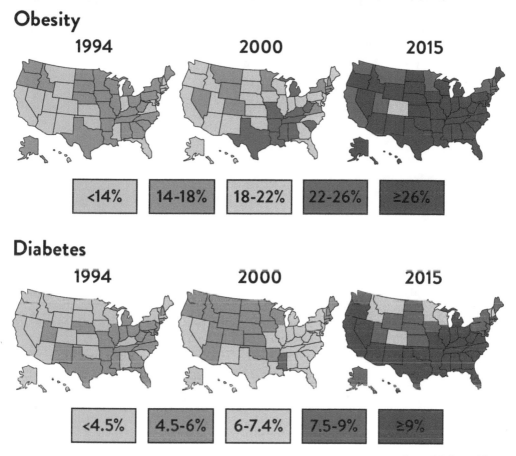

| 1994 | 2000 | 2015 |

| <14% | 14-18% | 18-22% | 22-26% | ≥26% |

## Diabetes

| 1994 | 2000 | 2015 |

| <4.5% | 4.5-6% | 6-7.4% | 7.5-9% | ≥9% |

www.cdc.gov/diabetes/data

You can take the following test and determine your risk for developing diabetes.

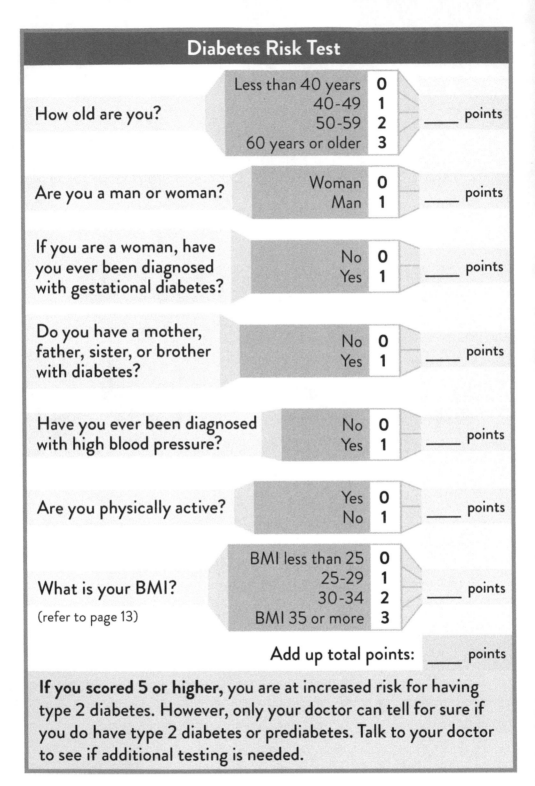

## Diabetes Risk Test

**How old are you?**

| | |
|---|---|
| Less than 40 years | 0 |
| 40-49 | 1 |
| 50-59 | 2 |
| 60 years or older | 3 |

_____ points

**Are you a man or woman?**

| | |
|---|---|
| Woman | 0 |
| Man | 1 |

_____ points

**If you are a woman, have you ever been diagnosed with gestational diabetes?**

| | |
|---|---|
| No | 0 |
| Yes | 1 |

_____ points

**Do you have a mother, father, sister, or brother with diabetes?**

| | |
|---|---|
| No | 0 |
| Yes | 1 |

_____ points

**Have you ever been diagnosed with high blood pressure?**

| | |
|---|---|
| No | 0 |
| Yes | 1 |

_____ points

**Are you physically active?**

| | |
|---|---|
| Yes | 0 |
| No | 1 |

_____ points

**What is your BMI?**

(refer to page 13)

| | |
|---|---|
| BMI less than 25 | 0 |
| 25-29 | 1 |
| 30-34 | 2 |
| BMI 35 or more | 3 |

_____ points

Add up total points: _____ points

**If you scored 5 or higher,** you are at increased risk for having type 2 diabetes. However, only your doctor can tell for sure if you do have type 2 diabetes or prediabetes. Talk to your doctor to see if additional testing is needed.

Diabetes is dangerous from a long-term perspective because high blood sugar levels can slowly damage arteries. There are two categories of vascular problems, called microvascular damage and macrovascular damage. Microvascular damage, as the name implies, happens at the level of the very tiny arterial branches within organs. These are the changes that lead to peripheral neuropathy, amputations, chronic kidney disease and retinal disease leading to blindness. Macrovascular damage occurs in the larger arteries, leading to the build-up of plaque, heart attacks, strokes and peripheral vascular disease, often involving the lower extremities. The risk for macrovascular complications actually starts to go up during the years of prediabetes.

Diabetes develops when the pancreas can no longer make enough insulin to compensate for the insulin resistance. For a long time the pancreas ramps up insulin production to compensate for the reduced capacity of cells to respond to the insulin signal. Eventually, the pancreas enters a burned out state and insulin production goes down. This is when blood sugar levels really start to shoot up. The key to diabetes prevention is to detect high risk individuals before pancreatic function starts to go down. By losing weight and exercising regularly, the insulin resistance can be reversed. A dramatic example of how even diabetes can sometimes be reversed is seen in patients who undergo bariatric surgery (surgery to reduce the size of the stomach or reduce the absorption of nutrients in the small intestine). With the extreme weight loss following the surgery, diabetes is reversed in a majority of these patients.

# How is my posture?

Poor posture places stress on the spine, the hips and the shoulders. Over the decades, it can lead to chronic back pain and arthritis. Poor posture also reduces the ability of the lungs to expand, thereby reducing gas exchange in the lungs. Poor posture also has an adverse effect on mood and confidence.

Correct posture should be maintained while sitting, standing and walking. The pelvis should be tilted forward, the spine should be straight, and the neck should be in line with the thoracic spine. The chin should be slightly tilted downwards. The shoulders should be relaxed, expanding the chest, and lowered. This posture allows for deep, relaxed breathing, a confident and youthful attitude, and increased energy.

To check your posture, have someone take pictures of you sitting and standing in your normal posture. You can also back up to a wall and see how easy and natural it is for you to have your hips, back and head touching the wall.

For help with developing good posture, visit the website of Esther Gokhale. She has studied people in many cultures and at many ages to discover the keys to a healthy back and healthy posture. Her book is called 8 Steps to a Pain Free Back. By following her program, you can regain the posture you naturally had as a child, strengthen key muscles involved in good posture, stretch out the spine, and reduce chronic back pain.

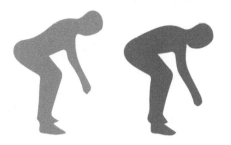

Bend at the hips, not waist

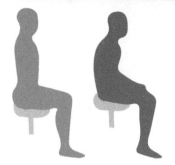

Keep your chest open and back straight

An anteverted pelvis facilitates healthy posture.

A retroverted pelvis leads to tense back muscles or slumping

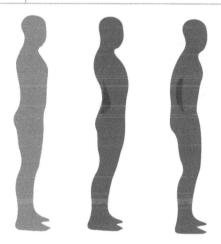

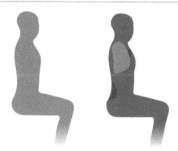

Relax your back and chest muscles to ease breathing in your chest and back rather than belly

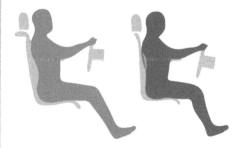

Use a cushion to stretch your back when you sit. Keep feet hip width and lengthen spine.

*Esther Gokhale*

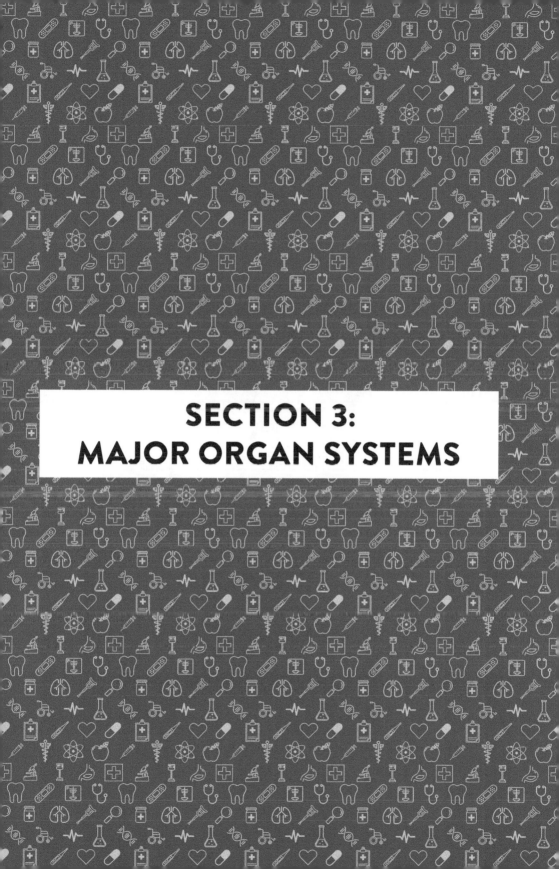

# SECTION 3:
# MAJOR ORGAN SYSTEMS

# How is my heart?

The heart is essentially a pump that delivers blood to the organs and tissues of the body. This is no easy task, as the requirements of each organ and tissue change from moment to moment. The amount of blood leaving the heart each minute is called the cardiac output. When we go from resting quietly to exercising rigorously, the cardiac output increases up to six-fold. Heart muscle never stops working. Assuming an average heart rate per day of 70, by the age of 50 the heart will have beaten (70 x 60 x 24 x 365 x 50) almost 2 billion times!

## Anatomy of the Heart

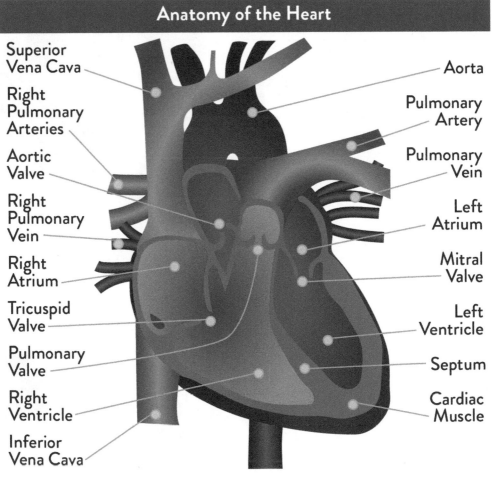

Superior Vena Cava

Right Pulmonary Arteries

Aortic Valve

Right Pulmonary Vein

Right Atrium

Tricuspid Valve

Pulmonary Valve

Right Ventricle

Inferior Vena Cava

Aorta

Pulmonary Artery

Pulmonary Vein

Left Atrium

Mitral Valve

Left Ventricle

Septum

Cardiac Muscle

In order for the heart to function appropriately, there has to be enough blood flow getting to the muscle (through the coronary arteries), the valves have to be opening and closing correctly, the conduction system has to be functioning well (the electrical signals that trigger muscle contraction), and the muscle itself has to be contracting normally and relaxing normally.

Heart attacks (myocardial infarction) occur when a plaque in the coronary arteries ruptures through the wall. This triggers a clot to form at the site of the rupture. If the clot is big enough, it can obstruct the artery. The sudden lack of blood flow to the dependent heart muscle (called ischemia) injures and can permanently damage the muscle. If the artery is opened quickly enough with a balloon and a stent, the muscle can be salvaged. When a large amount of muscle is damaged, the pump function of the heart is compromised and heart failure develops.

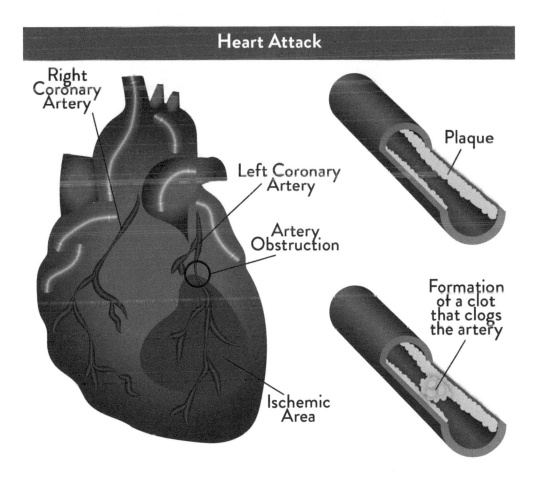

## Heart Attack

Right Coronary Artery

Left Coronary Artery

Artery Obstruction

Ischemic Area

Plaque

Formation of a clot that clogs the artery

Heart valves can develop leaks or become narrowed. Either situation can compromise heart function. Over time, if the heart has trouble compensating for the valve malfunction, heart failure will occur.

## Types of Valve Disease

### Stenosis

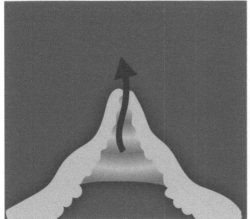

Valve doesn't open all the way, not enough blood passes through

### Regurgitation

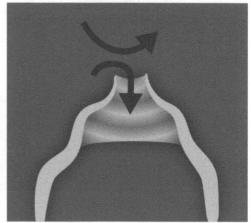

Valve doesn't close all the way, blood leaks backwards

The conduction system depends on a normal electrical signal initiated by the pacemaker tissue at the top of the heart called the sinus node. Sinus rhythm is the name given to the normal heart rhythm (controlled by the sinus node). Numerous conditions can arise where sinus rhythm is replaced by an abnormal rhythm. Abnormal fast rhythms are called tachycardias, Abnormal slow rhythms are called bradycardias. All the abnormal rhythms are grouped together under the heading arrhythmias. An electrocardiogram (ECG) is used to determine if the rhythm is normal or abnormal. The P wave indicates atrial, or upper chamber contraction. The QRS wave indicates ventricular, or lower chamber contraction. The T wave indicates repolarization, when the heart muscle returns from the depolarized to the resting state.

Typical symptoms that might indicate a problem with the heart include chest pain, shortness of breath, palpitations or lightheadedness. Chest pain is called angina when it is caused by inadequate blood flow to the heart muscle. Shortness of breath, also called dyspnea, could be caused by fluid build-up in the lungs from heart failure. Palpitations are usually associated with an arrhythmia. If cardiac output is severely compromised, such as with a very slow heart rate (bradycardia), lightheadedness or loss of consciousness (syncope) might occur.

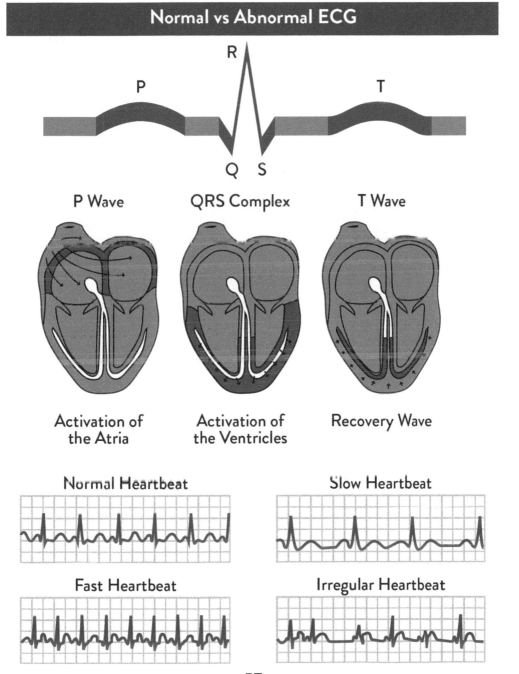

## Normal vs Abnormal ECG

P Wave
QRS Complex
T Wave

Activation of the Atria
Activation of the Ventricles
Recovery Wave

Normal Heartbeat
Slow Heartbeat

Fast Heartbeat
Irregular Heartbeat

If one or more of these symptoms are present, a comprehensive history and physical exam will provide enough information to determine what other diagnostic tests are necessary. For example, if the physical exam reveals a heart murmur, then an echocardiogram will reveal any problems with the heart valves.

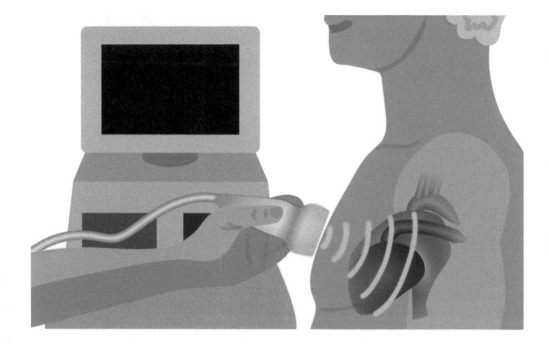

# How are my veins?

Veins begin after the arteries have released their oxygen to the tissues at the level of the capillaries. The veins travel back to the lungs with carbon dioxide, where gas exchange unloads the carbon dioxide and once again replenishes the blood with oxygen for the next circuit around the body. Veins contain one-way valves so that blood is constantly pushed towards the right side of the heart and from there to the lungs. There are two main categories of vein disease:

## Thrombosis (blood clots)

This occurs most commonly in the leg veins. Major risks factors include cancer, prolonged immobility, pregnancy, post-surgery, genetic tendencies and contraception use. A clot in a surface vein is called superficial thrombophlebitis, while a clot in a deep vein is called deep vein thrombosis (DVT). Only clots in the deep veins are dangerous, because they can break loose and travel to the lungs, thereby causing a pulmonary embolism, which is potentially fatal. Up to half of DVT's are asymptomatic. Symptoms may include calf pain, pain in the ball of the foot, calf tenderness and calf swelling. Diagnosis is made with an ultrasound test, and treatment is with anticoagulants for at least 6 months.

## Venous insufficiency

This occurs when the one-way valves in the veins no longer work correctly, leading to pooling of the blood. This leads to either superficial insufficiency, known as varicose veins, and deep vein insufficiency. Varicose veins are dilated, snake-like, and lie just below the skin. In addition to being unsightly, varicose veins can cause burning, aching or itching. They can occasionally lead to skin ulcers. Treatments include exercise, weight loss and compression stockings. When the deep veins are involved, chronic venous insufficiency can develop. This can actually be due to a prior DVT. Symptoms of chronic venous insufficiency include leg swelling, pain, darkened skin color and coarsening of the skin texture. Treatment includes compression stockings, leg elevation and possibly diuretics.

# How are my kidneys?

The kidneys do much more than just eliminate bodily wastes:

The kidneys help regulate blood pressure, convert inactive vitamin D to active vitamin D, produce a substance necessary for red blood cell production in the bone marrow, and are exquisitely sensitive to the amount of water in the body.

## What does the Kidney Do?

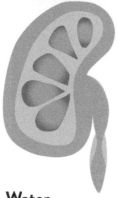

**Wastes**
Gets rid of urea, uric acid, toxins, and other wastes via urine

**Blood Pressure**
Makes sure that pressure isn't too high or too low

**Water**
Ensures that there's not too much or too little water in the body

**Heart**
Maintains a balance of electrolytes (like potassium, sodium, and calcium), which is critical for heart rhythm

**Blood**
Releases erythropoietin, which tells bone marrow to make red blood cells

**Bones**
Activates Vitamin D, which helps the body absorb calcium

**Acid-Base Balance**
Makes sure that the body isn't too acidic or too alkaline

Kidney disease tends to develop silently over many years. The most important risk factors are diabetes and hypertension. A blood test can measure the amount of urea (BUN or blood urea nitrogen) and creatinine in the blood. As kidney disease progresses, BUN and creatinine go higher and higher. If chronic kidney disease is discovered early, it is easier to prevent progression by treating the underlying risk factor, such as diabetes or hypertension.

Diabetes and hypertension are responsible for most cases of chronic kidney disease. If you have one or both of these conditions, it is important to periodically test for protein in the urine. In the very early stages of damage to the kidney, small amounts of a protein called albumin leak into the urine. This is called microalbuminuria. The presence of microalbuminuria is associated with a higher risk for cardiovascular disease and a higher risk for progression to more advanced stages of chronic kidney disease.

## Kidney Disease

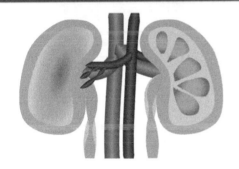

### Symptoms

Most people with moderate to severe kidney disease don't experience any symptoms

### Risk Factors

### Timeline

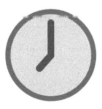

Early detection and treatment of kidney disease can slow the progression

Diabetes

High Blood Pressure

Genetics

Heart Disease

In fact, microalbuminuria is most likely caused by damage to the endothelium and other layers of the artery wall in the kidneys, thereby causing proteins to leak out of the artery. Both hypertension and diabetes are systemic diseases that damage the artery wall. High blood sugar and hypertension are both components of the metabolic syndrome, so it comes as no surprise that metabolic syndrome is also associated with microalbuminuria.

Chronic kidney disease does not cause pain, so the condition can worsen insidiously. Acute kidney disease comes on suddenly. Kidney stones form slowly, so are a chronic process, but when a stone completely obstructs the urinary system, it produces excruciating pain in the flank region, and becomes an acute problem. Infections in the bladder or kidney are also examples of an acute process, and may cause bleeding in the urine (hematuria) or a burning sensation. Kidney infections can also become systemic, causing fever and chills, and sometimes leading to sepsis.

# How is my respiratory tract?

The respiratory tract begins with the nose, extends down through the throat, and then continues into the trachea, which then branches into the lungs.

## The Respiratory System

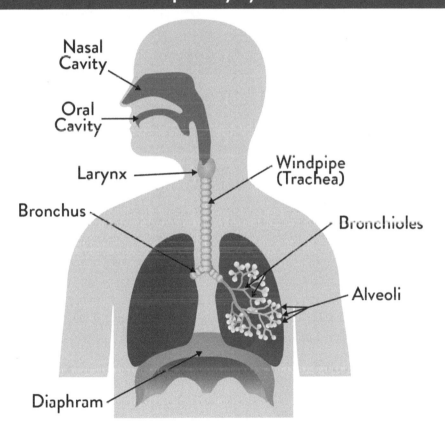

- Nasal Cavity
- Oral Cavity
- Larynx
- Bronchus
- Windpipe (Trachea)
- Bronchioles
- Alveoli
- Diaphram

Upper respiratory diseases are very common, and include colds, sore throats and sinus infections. Most of these are due to viral infections and are self-limiting. Antibiotics will only be helpful if there is a bacterial component to the infection (such as strep throat). Coughs can be productive or non-productive. A non-productive cough is dry and hacking. A productive cough results in the production of phlegm, either clear or purulent (yellow or green, sometimes with flecks of blood). Upper or lower respiratory infections can produce coughs. Bronchitis or pneumonia are examples of lower respiratory tract infections that usually cause productive coughs. These should always be evaluated by your physician. A chronic cough should also always be investigated, as it may be due to an underlying process such as a cancer or a chronic low-grade infection.

Coughing up blood is called hemoptysis. It may be due to an underlying infection or a cancer. It always requires careful evaluation to determine the cause.

Wheezing occurs when the bronchial tubes in the lungs constrict. This makes it more difficult for air to flow through the passageways, thus producing the high-pitched wheezing noise. Asthma causes acute constriction of the bronchi, often in response to an allergic stimulus. Bronchodilators are used to open up the airways. Severe asthma attacks can be life-threatening, and are treated with epinephrine injections. Wheezing should always be investigated and treated appropriately.

The lungs bring oxygen from the air into specialized sacs (alveoli) that permit diffusion of the oxygen into the blood stream during inspiration. Simultaneously, carbon dioxide diffuses out of the blood stream and is eliminated with expiration. So, breathing in and out we control the basic process of aerobic respiration, which uses oxygen to produce lots of energy in the form of ATP.

The lung diseases that are most common in middle and older age groups are chronic obstructive pulmonary disease (COPD, also called emphysema and chronic bronchitis), asthma, pneumonia, acute bronchitis, pulmonary emboli (blood clots in the lungs) and lung cancer. The most common symptoms of lung disease are shortness of breath, cough and chest pain.

Lung function is measured using a pulmonary function test (PFT). The subject takes as deep a breath as possible and then exhales the whole breath as fast as possible into the measuring apparatus. This allows the doctor to assess lung capacity (volume of air taken in during inspiration) and airway integrity (speed at which air leaves the lungs). The result is a flow/volume loop. Abnormal lung function can be restrictive (reduced volume) or obstructive (reduced flow speed).

# Normal & Abnormal FV Loops

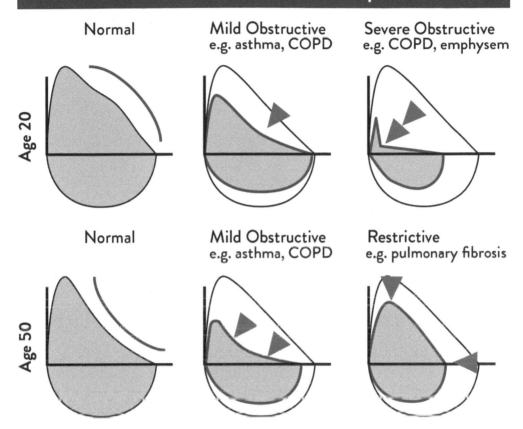

In the picture above, the horizontal axis is volume, typically in liters, and the vertical axis is flow, in liters/second. When flow is decreased, as in COPD, the flow loop is reduced in height. When volume is decreased, as in chronic fibrosis (loss of elasticity of lung tissue due to chronic inflammation), the loop is reduced in width. Lung volumes are also decreased in obesity, as the fat in the abdominal cavity interferes with normal lung expansion.

If you have symptoms or signs on physical exam of lung disease, then it may be necessary to obtain either a chest X-ray or a chest CT scan. Chest X-rays are used to diagnose pneumonia, fluid around the lungs (pleural effusion), heart failure and other conditions that change the appearance of the lungs. A chest CT has a much higher resolution than a chest X-ray. It can detect very small cancers, subtle changes to the bronchial tubes, and blood clots in the lungs (this diagnosis requires an angiogram to be done as part of the CT scan).

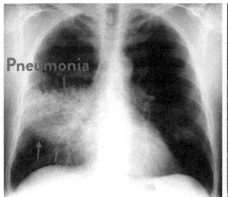 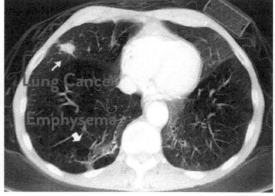

The picture on the left above is a chest X-ray showing a pneumonia in the right lung (arrows). The picture on the right is a chest CT scan showing a cancer (white circular mass), emphysema (areas that are black due to the destruction of lung tissue) and a cigarette pack!

# How is my liver?

The liver sits on the right side of the abdomen just below the diaphragm. It functions as the master metabolic organ of the body, and is crucial for energy metabolism, drug metabolism and protein metabolism.

## What does the Liver Do?

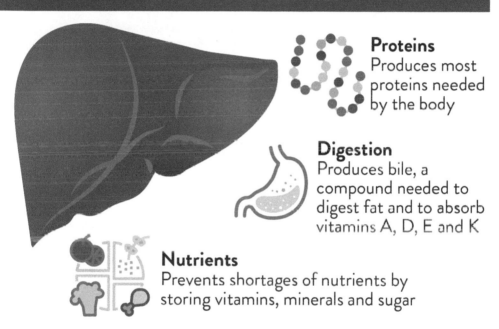

**Proteins**
Produces most proteins needed by the body

**Digestion**
Produces bile, a compound needed to digest fat and to absorb vitamins A, D, E and K

**Nutrients**
Prevents shortages of nutrients by storing vitamins, minerals and sugar

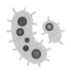

**Bacteria**
Helps the body fight infection by removing bacteria from the blood

**Food**
Metabolizes, or breaks down, nutrients from food to produce energy

**Blood**
Produces most of the substances that regulate blood clotting

**Toxins**
Removes potentially toxic byproducts of certain medications

Because the liver is the main organ charged with processing fats and sugars, it is very susceptible to the accumulation of fat when excess calories are consumed. The liver makes special particles- the VLDL particles- to send triglycerides out into the circulation for distribution to other parts of the body, such as muscle and fat cells. If too many triglycerides are made, the liver becomes overwhelmed and cannot make enough VLDL particles. In that situation, triglycerides accumulate inside the liver cells and cause chronic inflammation. This is called non-alcoholic fatty liver disease. It is becoming very common due to the prevalence of overweight and obese people.

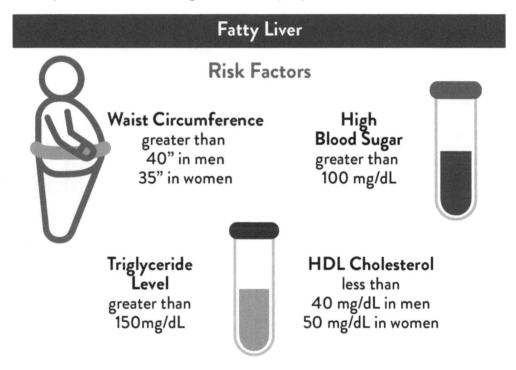

## Fatty Liver

### Risk Factors

**Waist Circumference**
greater than
40" in men
35" in women

**High
Blood Sugar**
greater than
100 mg/dL

**Triglyceride
Level**
greater than
150mg/dL

**HDL Cholesterol**
less than
40 mg/dL in men
50 mg/dL in women

If the chronic inflammation is severe enough, it can eventually lead to cirrhosis and liver failure. At Scripps Executive Health, we measure several liver enzymes in the blood that become elevated with liver inflammation.

The other major cause of chronic liver disease is alcoholic fatty liver disease. The liver converts alcohol to acetate which is then used to synthesize fatty acids. Again, if the liver cannot efficiently remove the triglycerides in VLDL particles, fatty liver develops, along with chronic inflammation. Anyone who consumes more than 1-2 alcoholic beverages per day is at risk for fatty liver disease.

## Symptoms

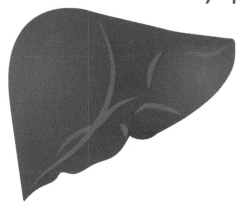

**None:** Fatty Liver Disease is often a silent killer because the disease progression is very slow and gradual. Many patients experience very few symptoms, leaving them unaware of their condition until it is critical.

## Causes

High Fat, Sugar or Carbohydrate Diet

Alcohol

Too Much Iron

Obesity

Certain Medications

Diabetes, High Blood Pressure, Cholesterol or Hepatitis

## Diagnosis

Medical history review and liver enzyme examination

Liver biopsy

Ultrasound and other tests: X-ray, MRI, FibroScan

Some people are missing important genes necessary for processing triglycerides. With too much alcohol, fats, or sugars in the diet, their blood triglycerides rise to dangerously high levels. When the blood triglycerides are consistently above 500 to 1000, pancreatitis can develop. This is another important piece of information obtained with the lipid panel.

# Treatment

### Change Eating Habits

reduce carbohydrates, fats and sugars, increase fruits and vegetables

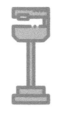

**Weight loss**

### Control Risk Factors

reduce cholesterol & blood pressure, control diabetes

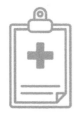

Annual checkups

**Be extra careful with medications or food supplements**

Avoid alcohol

Acute inflammatory liver disease is most often caused by viral infections. There are three common types of hepatitis, called A, B and C (two uncommon forms are D and E). Hepatitis A is caused by a virus transmitted in the feces of infected carriers, so someone with the disease who does not wash his or her hands well after a bowel movement may touch food then consumed by an unsuspecting victim. Hepatitis B requires contact with the infected body fluids of a carrier, via for example a shared needle or sexual intercourse. Hepatitis C also requires contact with body fluids. Both hepatitis B an C can convert from an acute to a chronic form. Chronic carriers may have no symptoms for many years, but eventually can develop end-stage liver disease or liver cancer. The most common symptoms of acute hepatitis are fatigue, dark urine, pale stools, yellow skin and eyes, and tenderness in the upper right abdomen.

Another cause of acute liver disease is gallstones. The gallbladder sits underneath the liver and stores bile acids for secretion into the intestine after a meal. Sometimes the bile solidifies into stones. Most of these stones are asymptomatic, but occasionally one will block the bile duct. This causes an obstruction which leads to inflammation and backing up of bile into the liver. Symptoms include intense pain in the right upper abdomen, fever, jaundice and nausea and vomiting. Sometimes symptoms will be more subtle, or wax and wane, for example if the stone only intermittently blocks the bile duct.

# How is my gastrointestinal tract?

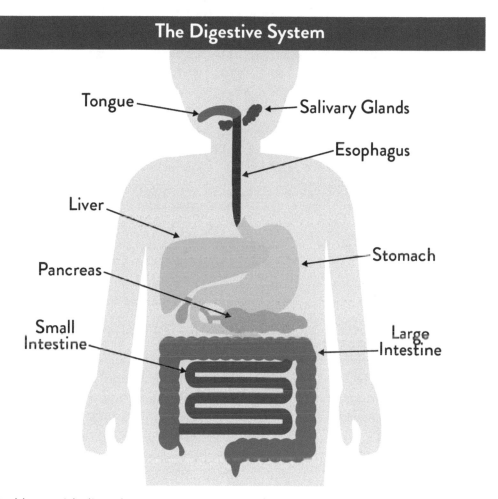

**The Digestive System**

- Tongue
- Salivary Glands
- Esophagus
- Liver
- Stomach
- Pancreas
- Small Intestine
- Large Intestine

Problems with digestion are very common. At the Center for Executive Health, the most frequent conditions we encounter are:

- Gastroesophageal reflux disease (GERD)
- Irritable bowel syndrome
- Peptic ulcer disease
- Chronic constipation
- Diverticulitis

GERD, or gastroesophageal reflux disease, is extremely common. About 60 million American adults experience the condition at least once a month. It can have a significant impact on quality of life, including enjoyment of food, sleep quality and work concentration. As the name implies, acids from the stomach back up into the esophagus, because the lower esophageal sphincter is not working properly. The term heartburn is often used to describe the symptoms. The lower esophagus can become chronically inflamed, which increases the long-term risk for esophageal cancer. Certain foods and beverages associated with GERD are chocolate, peppermint, fatty foods, coffee and alcohol. Symptoms can be improved by reducing food portion size, avoiding eating within 2-3 hours of going to bed, losing weight, elevating the head of the bed, and taking antacids or proton pump inhibitors (like Nexium, Prevacid and Prilosec).

Irritable Bowel Syndrome (IBS) affects 10-15% of adults in America. The cause is unknown, but many researchers suspect that disruptions to the brain-gut connection are involved. This results in abnormal colon motility, so that instead of gently contracting to move the gut contents (a process called peristalsis), the colon becomes hyperactive, with exaggerated contractions of the smooth muscles in the colon wall. This can lead to bouts of diarrhea, excessive gas, or even constipation. A network of 100 million neurons connects the intestine with the brain. This enteric nervous system has been called the body's second brain, because imbalances of neurotransmitters such as serotonin in the gut neurons can result in diarrhea (excessive serotonin secretion) or constipation (too little serotonin). Signals back and forth between the gut and the brain have a profound effect on the bowel environment. In addition, poor diets, or diets that are poorly tolerated for genetic reasons, can disrupt the microbiome, the billions of bacteria residing in the colon. Finally, small intestine bacterial overgrowth (SIBO) is another potential cause for chronic GI distress.

The GI tract has extensive immune system components, and microbiome disorders can trigger inflammation, which in turn can have effects on the immune system elsewhere throughout the body. The gut immune system is called gut-associated lymphoid tissue, or GALT. Much research is currently being done in this area to determine exactly how the gut microbes interact with the gut immune system, and how this may be implicated in IBS, inflammatory bowel disease, leaky gut syndrome and even colon cancer.

Peptic ulcer disease occurs when a bacteria called H. Pylori destroys the protective lining in the stomach or duodenum, leading to an erosion of the wall, abdominal pain, and sometimes dangerous bleeding at the site of the ulcer. Up to half the population harbors H. Pylori but only a small fraction of those who carry the bacteria actually develop ulcers. Other conditions that can interact with the bacteria and possibly trigger ulcer formation include chronic aspirin use, chronic NSAID use (non-steroidal anti-inflammatory drugs such as Motrin), cigarettes, and alcohol.

As we mentioned above, IBS is a potential cause of constipation due to abnormal motility of the colon. Chronic constipation can also be caused by a diet low in fiber, physical inactivity and certain drugs (opioids, antidepressants, anticonvulsants, calcium channel blockers, aluminum-containing antacids, and diuretics). Aging slows down intestinal transit, which causes more water to be absorbed from the stool. Inadequate fluid intake can also harden the stools. Changes to daily routine, such as travel, can also disrupt the circadian rhythms that control bowel movements.

A low fiber diet is also implicated in the development of diverticulosis, which is a condition defined by the presence of small herniated pouches throughout the colon. The bowel wall protrudes through the smooth muscle layer of the colon to form the pouches. If a pouch gets infected, it can cause diverticulitis. Harmful bacteria grow in the pouch and trigger an acute inflammatory process that can be mild, with only local pain, usually left upper quadrant of the abdomen, or can be severe, with development of peritonitis. 80-85% of patients with diverticulosis will remain asymptomatic. About 5% develop diverticulitis, and of those, 15-25% will have severe enough disease to warrant surgery.

Colon cancer is, unfortunately, often asymptomatic until its later stages. Key facts include:

- In 2017, there were 135,000 new cases and 50,000 deaths
- It's the second leading cause of cancer deaths in the US
- 90% of cases are in people over the age of 50
- If you have a first degree relative with colon cancer, your risk is two to three times higher than average
- 60% of colon cancer deaths are preventable with appropriate screening
- Screening methods include colonoscopy, fecal occult blood test, fecal immune chemical test (FIT) and stool DNA test

# How is my prostate?

The prostate gland produces the fluid component of sperm. It sits below the bladder and around the urethra (the tubular structure that carries urine from the bladder through the penis). As men age, the prostate tissue can enlarge, through a process called hypertrophy. The risk factors for prostate hypertrophy (called BPH for benign prostatic hypertrophy) are family history of the condition, ethnicity (less common in Asians than in white and black men), some forms of heart disease, use of beta blocker and diabetes.

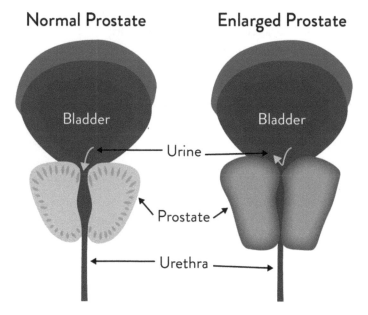

As the urethra gets compressed by the enlarging prostate, it becomes more difficult to completely empty the bladder. Symptoms of the condition include reduced force of the urinary stream and more frequent urination, including having to get up during the night.

As part of a comprehensive physical exam, the size of the prostate can be evaluated. If it is found to be enlarged, there are both herbal and pharmaceutical options for shrinking its size.

Prostate cancer is very common. The blood test used to screen for it is called the PSA test, for prostate specific antigen. Unfortunately, there is much controversy concerning the interpretation of the PSA results. Typically, the cut point for an abnormal test is 4 ng/mL. But studies have shown that some men with lower levels can have prostate cancer and many men with abnormal levels do not have cancer but may be subjected to biopsies. Prostatitis, an inflammation of the prostate, can also raise the PSA level. As a general rule, the higher the PSA, the more likely cancer is present. About 25% of men who undergo a biopsy due to an elevated PSA will have prostate cancer. But many of those cancers are slow growing and will never pose a risk. A large study showed that even though PSA screening detected more prostate cancers than in a comparable population that did not undergo screening (called the control group), the rate of deaths from prostate cancer was the same in both groups.

- 1 in 7 men will be diagnosed with prostate cancer
- 60% are age 65 or older
- 90% with localized cancer will live 5 years or more after diagnosis
- There are 2.9 million prostate cancer survivors in the US
- Prostate cancer is the number 2 cause of cancer deaths in men after lung cancer

# How are my breasts?

During puberty, female hormones trigger breast development, or mammogenesis. A complex branching system of ducts develops, along with expansion of fat and connective tissue. During pregnancy, further breast growth occurs in preparation for lactation and breast-feeding. Because the female breast is more complex than the male breast, most common breast conditions occur much more frequently in females.

The most common breast condition is fibrocystic disease, also called benign proliferative breast disease. It occurs in up to 40% of women. Clinical symptoms, such as pain and tenderness, occur in about 10% of women. The condition is rare after menopause. The cause is unknown, but may be related to hormonal imbalances. Breast tissue feels firm and rubbery, with occasionally palpable cysts and with intermittent tenderness. The condition can make it more difficult to palpate early breast cancer, and can make mammograms more challenging to read. There is a two-fold increased risk for cancer.

15-20% of women will develop benign breast lesions which may be cystic (fluid-filled) or solid. The presence of abnormal breast tissue can make it more likely that a false positive result will occur during mammography screening for breast cancer. For every breast cancer diagnosed, there are three to four false diagnoses, which may lead to unnecessary biopsies and may influence women to put off their next mammogram.

About 10% of women develop breast cancer, and a new case is diagnosed every 3 minutes in the US. Warning signs include:

- Breast skin puckering
- A lump in the breast or armpit
- Nipple discharge
- Dimpling of the nipple or nipple retraction

Breast cancer is the 2nd leading cause of cancer death in women, after lung cancer, but survival rates have tripled in the last 60 years. Two thirds of cases are in women 55 or older.

Risk factors include:

- Age
- Genetics (for example the BRCA1 and BRCA2 genes)
- Being overweight or obese
- Being white (although black women are more likely to get more aggressive forms of breast cancer)
- Having more than one alcoholic beverage per day

## What You Can Do

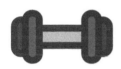

### Exercise

1.5 - 3 hours
of exercise a day
can lower your
risk by 30%

### Drink Less

Limit your alcohol
intake to 1 drink
or less per day

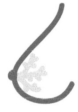

### Know the Signs

Know your own
breasts and what's
normal for you
and know what
is worrisome

Foods which may have some anti-cancer properties include:

- Pomegranates
- Grape seed extract
- Blueberries
- Curcumin

# How are my ovaries and uterus?

The female reproductive system consists of the ovaries, fallopian tubes and uterus, as well as the external genitalia.

The ovaries store eggs, and release one during ovulation (about 400 are released during the reproductive years). The ovaries also make the major female hormones- estrogen and progesterone.

The major disorders that can affect the ovaries include:

## Polycystic ovary syndrome (PCOS)

PCOS affects 10% of women during the reproductive years, but up to 50% may not know they have it. It is due to an excess secretion of male hormones (androgens). Symptoms may include abnormal body hair, weight gain, acne and infertility (it's the leading cause of infertility in women). PCOS is associated with insulin resistance and pre-diabetes. Obesity is a risk factor for insulin resistance. With insulin resistance, insulin levels rise and may boost androgen levels.

## Ovarian cysts

These are fluid-filled sacs that develop inside the ovary. They may cause pain in the abdomen or pelvis. A ruptured ovarian cyst typically causes severe pain and internal bleeding which is one-sided and sudden in onset.

Key facts about ovarian cancer:

- **Genetic risk associated with BRCA genes**
- **No test for early detection**
- **70% not discovered until stage 3 or 4**
- **Higher risk in women who have never been pregnant**
- **5th most common cancer in women**

The uterus provides a home for the fertilized egg while it develops into a fetus. Some common disorders include:

## Endometriosis

about 1 in 10 women of reproductive age suffer from the condition, which involves the growth of uterine tissue outside the uterus. Symptoms include infertility, painful sex, bleeding between periods, excessive pain and bleeding during periods, pelvic pain and fatigue. The main treatment options are surgery, hormones and pain medications.

## Fibroids

These are non-cancerous growths inside the uterus. They may cause pain and bleeding.

## Excessive bleeding during menstruation

Treatments include birth control pills and endometrial ablation, if symptoms are severe and persistent.

### Key Facts About Menopause

 Usually begins between the ages of 40 and 58 (average age 51) and is official after 12 months without a menstrual period

 Risk of cardiovascular disease rises rapidly after menopause

 Risk for osteoporosis doubles after menopause

 Symptoms vary in severity, but may include hot flashes, night sweats, insomnia, forgetfulness, reduced libido, mood swings, anxiety, vaginal dryness, incontinence and headaches

 There are both natural and hormonal treatments for the condition

# How is my thyroid?

The thyroid gland produces hormones (called T3 and T4) that help control the rates of metabolism in many tissues throughout the body. The hormones can speed up heart rate, raise body temperature, increase energy level, burn fat, increase digestive function, regulate cholesterol levels, influence menstruation and much more. The body sends signals to the brain to help regulate thyroid hormone levels.

## Hypothalamic-Pituitary-Thyroid Axis

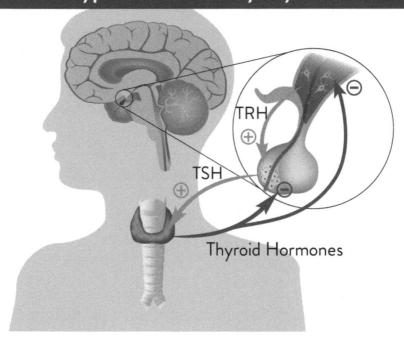

This is a classic example of a feedback loop. If thyroid hormone levels are high, the hypothalamus secretes less thyroid releasing hormone which in turn tells the pituitary to secrete less TSH (thyroid stimulating hormone). Conversely, if thyroid hormone levels are low, more TSH is secreted, telling the thyroid to make more thyroid hormones.

Low thyroid hormone levels can be caused by inadequate iodine in the diet, as iodine is an important element in the structure of T3 and T4. Autoimmune disease can cause either hypo or hyperthyroidism.

Thyroid nodules are very common, and are sometimes found on physical exam, or by imaging the thyroid with ultrasound. A small percentage of nodules secrete excessive thyroid hormone and cause hyperthyroidism. Most nodules do not produce thyroid hormone, and a small percentage of these are cancerous.

At Scripps Executive Health, we measure TSH to screen for abnormal thyroid function. Symptoms of hypothyroidism include fatigue, depression, cold intolerance, joint and muscle pain and insomnia. Symptoms of hyperthyroidism include increased irritability and anxiety, palpitations, tremor and heat intolerance.

# How are my eyes?

Aging brings with it the risk for several types of eye disease. The most common one is cataracts. Cataracts develop when the proteins in the lens start to clump together, losing their normal structure. Instead of being translucent, the lens gradually turns cloudy. Initially, the changes to vision are quite subtle. But as the lens becomes more opaque, less light can reach the retina, and symptoms worsen. About 22 million Americans over the age of 40 have cataracts. Cataract surgery involves removing the defective lens and replacing it with an artificial one. This restores normal vision.

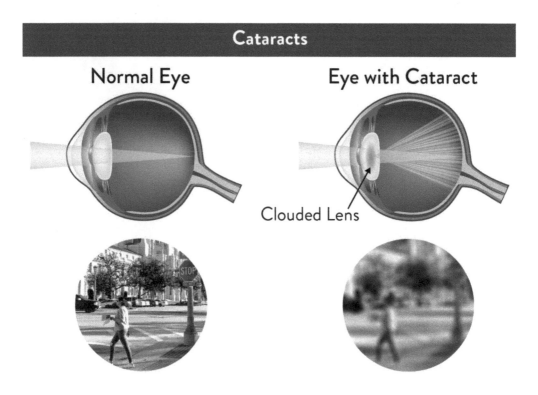

**Cataracts**

**Normal Eye**

**Eye with Cataract**

Clouded Lens

The next most common eye disease is macular degeneration. Over 10 million Americans have this condition and it is the leading cause of blindness in

America. The macula is the central region of the retina. When it degenerates, there is loss of the central field of vision. The disease is slowly progressive, gradually affecting many everyday skills such as reading, driving and recognizing faces.

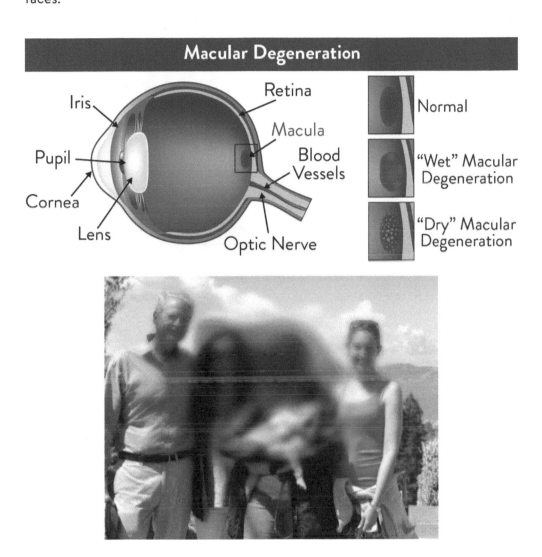

## Macular Degeneration

Iris
Retina
Macula
Pupil
Blood Vessels
Cornea
Lens
Optic Nerve

Normal

"Wet" Macular Degeneration

"Dry" Macular Degeneration

Unlike cataracts, for which there is a surgical procedure, and glaucoma, which can be stabilized with medications, macular degeneration is relentlessly progressive. Therefore it is important to do everything possible to help prevent its onset and progression. Diets high in fruits and vegetables are protective, while high saturated fat diets may increase risk. Fish and fish oil supplements may reduce risk. The following supplements are sometimes included in a single supplement for eye health:

- Vitamin C 500mg
- Vitamin E 400 IU
- Zinc 80mg
- Copper 2mg
- Lutein 10mg
- Zeaxanthin 2mg

Lutein and zeaxanthin are carotenoids (plant pigments with yellow, red and orange hues). Their protective effect in preventing eye disease may be related to their ability to absorb potentially damaging blue light. Here is a list of vegetables that contain them (egg yolks are also a good source):

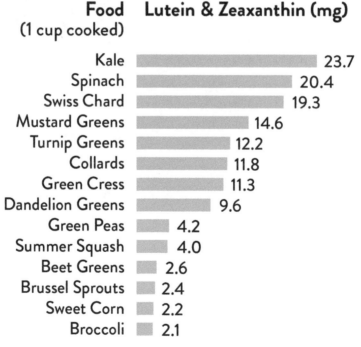

## Vegetables That Are Good For Your Eyes

| Food (1 cup cooked) | Lutein & Zeaxanthin (mg) |
|---|---|
| Kale | 23.7 |
| Spinach | 20.4 |
| Swiss Chard | 19.3 |
| Mustard Greens | 14.6 |
| Turnip Greens | 12.2 |
| Collards | 11.8 |
| Green Cress | 11.3 |
| Dandelion Greens | 9.6 |
| Green Peas | 4.2 |
| Summer Squash | 4.0 |
| Beet Greens | 2.6 |
| Brussel Sprouts | 2.4 |
| Sweet Corn | 2.2 |
| Broccoli | 2.1 |

*USDA National Nutrient Database for Standard Reference, Release 22 (2009)*

The third most common eye problem is glaucoma. In this condition, there is a gradual build-up of pressure inside the eye that compresses the optic nerve and can eventually lead to blindness. A special test called tonometry can measure the pressure in the eye. If it is increased, we refer you to an ophthalmologist for a more in-depth examination.

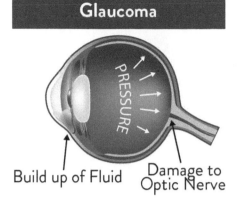

## Glaucoma

PRESSURE

Build up of Fluid

Damage to Optic Nerve

# How is my hearing?

Hearing loss is the third most common health problem in the US, after cardiovascular disease and arthritis.

## Hearing Loss in America

**1 in 3**
People over 60
have Hearing Loss

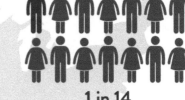

**1 in 14**
Gen X-ers already
have Hearing Loss

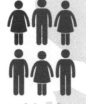

**1 in 6**
Baby Boomers
have Hearing Loss

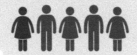

**1 in 5**
Teenagers have
some Hearing Loss

There are three types of hearing loss:

Outer Ear     Middle Ear     Inner Ear

Conductive    Sensorineural
Hearing Loss    Hearing Loss

Mixed Hearing Loss

Although there are many potential causes for hearing loss, the most common are age-related and excessive noise exposure.

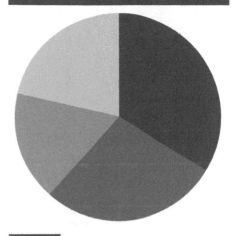

## Causes of Hearing Loss

At Scripps we check hearing using a special booth that isolates the client from outside noise. Sounds of increasing intensity and different frequencies are randomly generated. The client presses a button when he/she hears a sound. The final report looks something like this:

**33.7%** Loud Noises
**28%** Age
**17.1%** Infection/Injury
**16.8%** Other
**4.4%** Born with Hearing Loss

*League for Hard of Hearing*

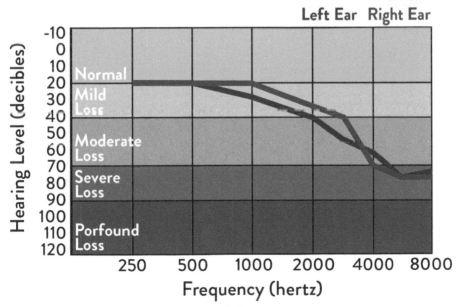

## Audiogram

Left Ear   Right Ear

Hearing Level (decibels)

-10
0
10   Normal
20
30   Mild
40   Loss
50   Moderate
60   Loss
70
80   Severe
90   Loss
100
110  Porfound
120  Loss

250   500   1000   2000   4000   8000

Frequency (hertz)

If a significant loss is noted, recommendations are made for follow-up with a specialist in hearing disorders. Because hearing loss can occur very gradually, many people remain undiagnosed and untreated for many years. This can have a significant effect on other serious conditions, as noted in the graphic below.

## Risks of Hearing Loss

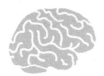 People with hearing loss experience a 30-40% faster decline in cognitive abilities compared to peers without hearing loss

 **90-95%** of people with hearing loss can be treated with hearing aids

 There is a significant association between high blood pressure and untreated hearing loss

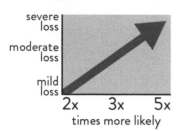 Adults with untreated hearing loss are more likely to develop dementia

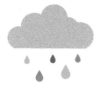 Adults with untreated hearing loss are more likely to report depression, anxiety and paranoia than peers who wear hearing aids

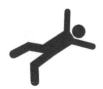 People with mild hearing loss are **3x** more likely to have a history of falling

# How is my musculoskeletal system?

The musculoskeletal system is made up of our bones and the soft tissues that are connected to the bones. The soft tissues, called tendons, muscles and ligaments, are encapsulated by myofascial tissue, a kind of connective tissue that is mesh-like and continuous throughout our body. Injuries can occur to any of these components of the musculoskeletal system. Injuries can be acute, due to a sudden explosive force, or chronic, due to repetitive small insults that lead to chronic inflammation and eventual permanent damage. Chronic back pain is the classic example of the latter. If you are experiencing chronic pain in the musculoskeletal system it is important to identify the underlying cause.

Very often, the pain is a consequence of a sedentary lifestyle, with poor joint mobility and inadequate muscle strength, or is the result of an injury that was never properly treated. Anti-inflammatory and analgesic medications can provide short-term relief but can be dangerous in the long-term, potentially damaging the kidneys, the liver or the stomach lining. Nonsteroidal anti-inflammatory drugs (NSAIDs) have even been shown to be associated with an increased risk for heart attacks when taken in high doses for extended periods.

Obesity causes systemic chronic low grade inflammation and puts extra stress on muscles and joints. A sedentary lifestyle also causes deterioration of muscle/tendon strength. Lack of exercise and daily activity also reduces joint mobility and muscle/tendon flexibility. At Scripps, we assess all components of the musculoskeletal system and recommend specific exercises and stretches for particular problem areas. We also recommend massage therapy and yoga as excellent modalities for improving musculoskeletal health. Myofascial release techniques can also be very effective at breaking up inflammation and scarring in the fascia surrounding the muscles.

Arthritis is the leading cause of disability in the US. Chronic joint inflammation eventually destroys the joint cartilage. Rheumatoid arthritis is an autoimmune disease, while osteoarthritis is caused by inflammation related to age, obesity, prior injury or prior overuse of a joint. A third type of arthritis is caused by elevated levels of uric acid that can crystallize in the joint spaces, triggering gout. Genetic factors also play an important role, as does sitting and standing posture.

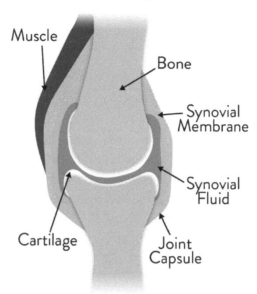

**Normal Joint**

Muscle

Bone

Synovial Membrane

Synovial Fluid

Cartilage

Joint Capsule

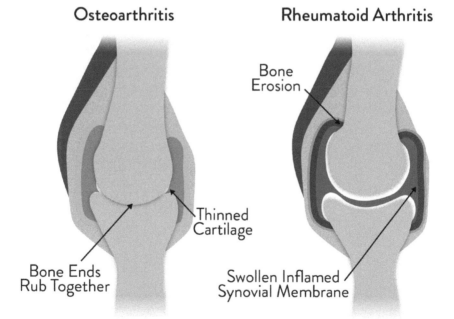

**Osteoarthritis**

Thinned Cartilage

Bone Ends Rub Together

**Rheumatoid Arthritis**

Bone Erosion

Swollen Inflamed Synovial Membrane

Over the age of 65, 1 in 2 Americans are diagnosed with some form of arthritis, predominantly osteoarthritis. Many of these cases can be prevented. Being overweight or obese puts extra stress on the joints, triggering inflammation. Low grade inflammation throughout the body is also more common in obesity.

Diets high in saturated fats and certain vegetable fats, such as corn oil, are pro-inflammatory, while diets high in fish oil, olive oil and fruits and vegetables tend to be anti-inflammatory. A program of regular stretching can keep the joints from stiffening. Regular exercise releases anti-inflammatory molecules post-exercise that help to rejuvenate body tissues. Standing correctly and sitting correctly prevents excessive stress on the spine.

Osteoporosis affects 1 in 2 women over the age of 50 and 1 in 4 men. Over 50 million Americans have the disease. Bone tissue is constantly being broken down and rebuilt by cells called osteoclasts and osteoblasts. As we age, the osteoblasts make less new bone, while the osteoclasts continue to break bone down.

## Normal Bone          Osteoporosis

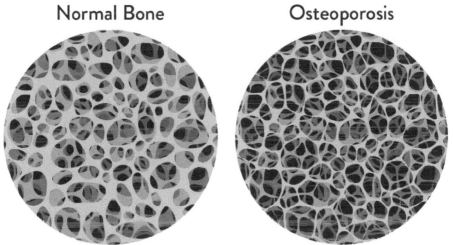

This eventually reduces bone density. The less dense bone is more susceptible to fractures. In the spine, this can cause compression fractures. In the hips, a fairly minor fall could result in a fracture if the bone is osteoporotic. Up to age 25 or 30, our bones increase in density, particularly in the setting of a calcium-rich diet and plenty of exercise. Then bone density gradually decreases. Factors that increase the risk for osteoporosis include menopause, low intake of calcium, inadequate vitamin D level, hyperthyroidism, chronic use of steroids, sedentary lifestyle, cigarette smoking and excessive alcohol consumption.

Carefully done studies to analyze the effectiveness of increasing calcium intake, either through supplements or increased low fat dairy products, have not been able to demonstrate any reduction in fracture risk. Calcium supplements have been implicated in an increased risk for heart attacks, although the data is somewhat controversial. They may also increase risk for kidney stones.

# How is my skin?

Our skin serves many functions in addition to protecting the internal organs from the surrounding environment. Sweat has molecules that can break down dangerous bacteria. Nerve endings react to heat, cold, pressure and vibration. Myriad blood vessels can constrict or dilate to help control internal temperature. Skin protects against excessive evaporation of water. Vitamin D is synthesized in the skin following exposure to sunlight.

Scripps Center for Executive Health includes an exam by a dermatologist. The most important aspect of the exam is to identify any lesions that are suspicious for skin cancer and perform a biopsy if indicated. There are three types of skin cancer as shown in the visual.

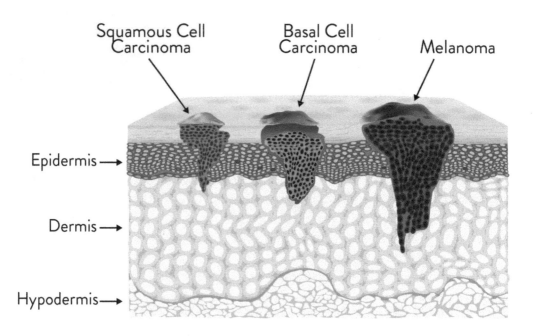

Squamous Cell Carcinoma | Basal Cell Carcinoma | Melanoma

Epidermis →

Dermis →

Hypodermis →

| Types of Skin Cancer | | |
| --- | --- | --- |
| Basal Cell | Squamous Cell | Melanoma |
| **Rank** | | |
| Most Common form of skin cancer | Second most common skin cancer | <2% of skin cancer cases |
| **Location** | | |
| In areas exposed to the sun | Sometimes spreads to other body parts | Can develop as a new or in a preexisting mole |
| **Treatment** | | |
| Rarely spreads Very rarely fatal | Almost all cases are curable | Causes the most skin cancer deaths |
| **Person** | | |
| Anyone - people with fair skin, blonde or red hair, light eyes | Usually age 50+ Majority of skin cancer in black people are squamous cell | One of the most common cancers in people younger than 30 |

The most important one to catch early is melanoma, as it can easily spread to other parts of the body. Only 1% of skin cancers are melanomas, but they are responsible for most of the mortality associated with skin cancers. The most important risk factors for skin cancer are having very fair skin and sun exposure, particularly exposure that results in sunburns. The graphic on the following page describes some of the features of melanomas.

Normal  Cancer

## Asymmetry

If you draw a line through the middle of the mole, the halves of a melanoma won't match in size.

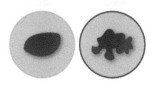

## Border

The edges of an early melanoma tend to be uneven, crusty or notched.

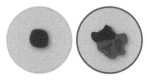

## Color

Healthy moles are uniform in color. A variety of colors, especially white and/or blue, is bad.

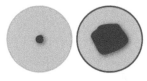

## Diameter

Melanomas are usually larger in diameter than a pencil eraser, although they can be smaller.

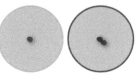

## Evolving

When a mole changes in size, shape or color, or begins to bleed or scab, this points to danger.

The other major category of skin problems are rashes. There are so many kinds of rashes that often a dermatologist is needed to make the correct diagnosis. Here are some of the most common rashes and their causes:

## Dermatitis (Eczema)

An ongoing condition that appears as patches of itchy or inflamed skin periodically and then subsides.

**Treatments:** Creams & Lotions

**Avoid:** Harsh soaps and detergents

# Rosacea

A chronic inflamatory skin condition that occurs periodically and appears similar to acne.

Appearance: Small red or pus-filled dots

Triggers: Sun exposure, extreme temperatures, skin products, certain foods

# Intertrigo

Intertrigo is inflammation caused by skin-to-skin friction, typically in warm, moist areas.

Treatments: Wear loosefitting clothing and use powders to reduce friction

# Psoriasis

A common skin condition that speeds up the life cycle of skin cells causing them to build up rapidly on the surface of the skin.

Appearance: Red patches of skin covered with thick, silvery scales or dry, cracked skin that may bleed

Treatments: There is no cure for psoriasis, but you can manage symptoms through lifestyle changes like managing stress and by using lotions

# Drug Rash

A side effect of a drug or an allergic reaction to medication. It begins as red spots that spread, covering large areas of the body.

Triggers: Common offenders are anti seizure drugs, antibiotics, and water pills (diuretics)

# Heat Rash (Miliaria)

When sweat is hindered, usually due to hot/humid weather, tight-fitting clothing, or overdressing, it can cause a heat rash.

Appearance: Small stinging red or clear fluid-filled bumps

Treatments: Wear loose, lightweight clothing and avoid excessive heat and humidity

## Shingles (Herpes Zoster)

Caused by the reactivation of the chickenpox virus, outbreaks start with itching or pain followed by groups of small blisters within a few days.

**Treatments:** Antiviral drugs may lessen the pain

## Poison Ivy

The leaves, roots and stems of poison ivy, poison oak, and poison sumac contain urushiol, an oily resin that can cause allergic rashes if it comes in contact with skin.

**Treatments:** Use a cold compress, calamine lotion, non-prescription hydrocortisone cream, or an antihistamine to ease itching

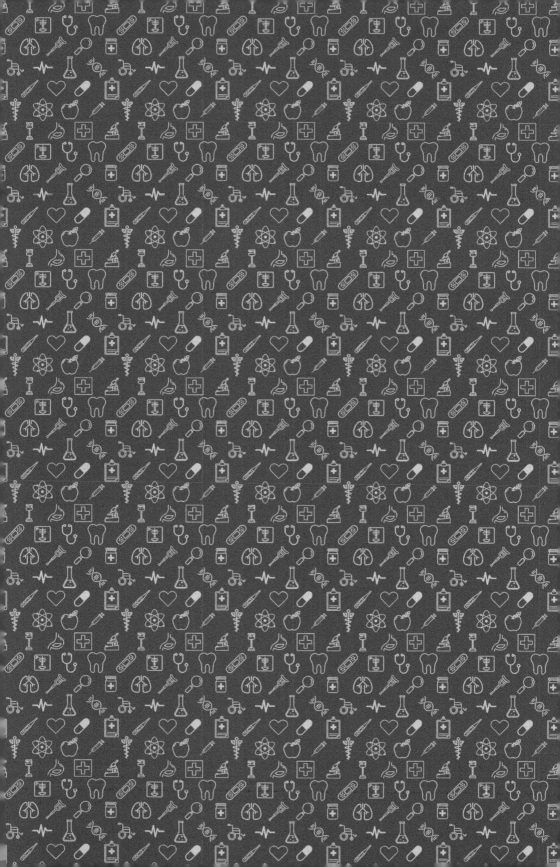

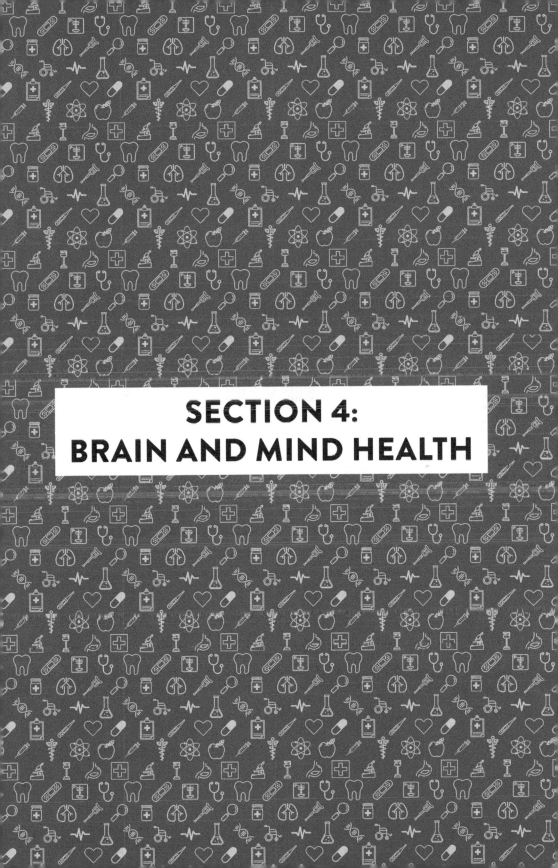

# SECTION 4:
# BRAIN AND MIND HEALTH

# How is my nervous system?

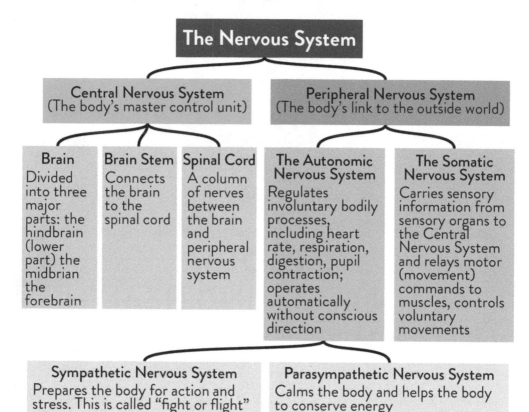

The central nervous system (CNS) is made up of the brain and the spinal cord (as opposed to the peripheral nervous system (PNS), which is made up of neurons that either originate or terminate in synapses with the spinal cord neurons descending from the brain). The most common causes of CNS disease are strokes (cerebrovascular accident or CVA), degenerative diseases of the brain such as Parkinson's disease and Alzheimer's disease, autoimmune diseases such as multiple sclerosis, and tumors, either benign, such as glioma, or malignant, such as glioblastoma.

Diagnosis of CNS disease requires a very careful analysis of symptoms and physical signs. For example, headaches are among the most common problems encountered in a general medicine practice. Around 45 million Americans suffer from chronic headaches. Most are caused by stress (tension headache), a significant percentage are migraines, some are related to sinus disease, and a very few are symptoms of brain tumors or expanding arterial aneurysms (an aneurysm is a section of artery with a weak wall that bulges outward and is at risk of rupturing). Tension headaches are usually mild to moderate in intensity and respond to analgesics such as aspirin or ibuprofen. Migraines are intensely painful and may be accompanied by nausea and vomiting and extreme sensitivity to light. Headaches from a severe underlying CNS condition such as a tumor or an aneurysm will often be accompanied by other neurological signs, such as visual symptoms, weakness, numbness, or unilateral hearing loss. Any headache that lasts longer than several days or that is of severe intensity should be evaluated by your physician, and may require diagnostic testing, such as a head CT scan or an MRI scan.

Numbness and tingling in an extremity may be a sign of CNS or PNS disease. If it is in a single extremity, such as an arm or a leg, it may be due to a nerve impingement syndrome, where the nerve exiting the spinal column is compressed by one of the vertebral bones. This could be due to a collapsed vertebra, a narrowing of the spinal column (spinal stenosis) or a bony spur caused by osteoarthritis. Disc herniation (discs are soft tissue structures between the vertebral bones) can also press on nerves and cause both back pain

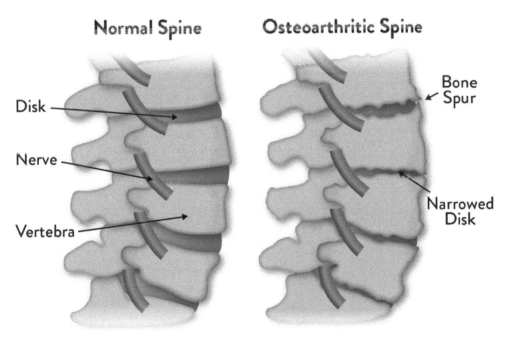

and tingling in the extremity served by the nerve. If the numbness and tingling is present in more than one extremity, it could be related to a a condition called peripheral neuropathy. This is a sign of damage to the PNS neurons. The most common cause of such a neuropathy is diabetes.

### Ischemic Stroke

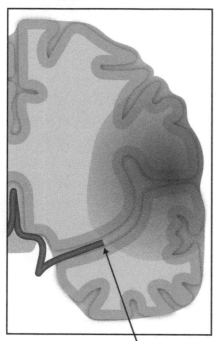

A clot blocks blood flow
to an area of the brain

### Hemorrhagic Stroke

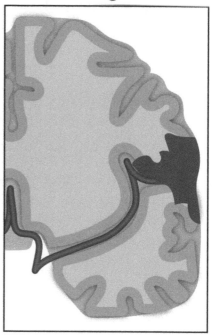

Bleeding occurs inside
or around brain tissue

A stroke or cerebrovascular accident (CVA) is caused by a blood clot blocking an artery to a part of the brain or by a ruptured artery bleeding into the brain. By far the most common type is the blood clot blocking an artery. The clot can originate from a plaque rupture in the carotid artery or one of the other arteries going to the brain, or it could form in the left atrium of the heart when a person is in a rhythm called atrial fibrillation. The symptoms of the stroke depend upon the artery that is blocked or bleeding. Common symptoms are one-sided weakness, a facial droop, trouble talking, or one-sided visual changes. Once symptoms occur, a narrow window of opportunity exists to prevent permanent damage. If the patient can get to an emergency room within 2 hours, an IV medication called a thrombolytic agent can be administered to try and dissolve the clot. Alternatively a special type of catheter can be threaded up into the artery with the clot and the clot can be removed. If done quickly enough, the brain tissue can be saved, and the symptoms will suddenly resolve.

## Parkinson's Disease

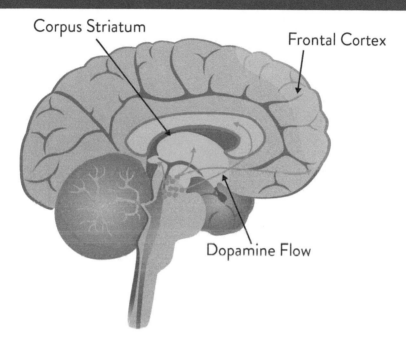

Corpus Striatum

Frontal Cortex

Dopamine Flow

**Normal Neuron**

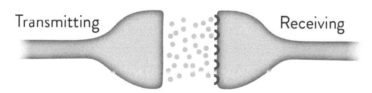

Transmitting

Receiving

**Neuron Affected by Parkinson's**

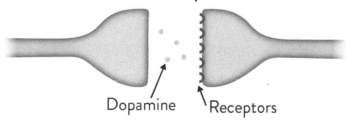

Dopamine

Receptors

Parkinson's disease is the second most common degenerative brain disease after Alzheimer's disease. It affects about a million people in America, with 50,000 new cases diagnosed a year. It typically occurs after the age of 60. The two most common symptoms are tremors and muscle rigidity. It is caused by the gradual destruction of neurons in a part of the brain called the substancia nigra. These cells produce a neurotransmitter called dopamine. The cause of the disease is unknown, although some cases have a genetic component and some cases may be caused by exposure to certain toxins.

# Am I showing any signs of Alzheimer's disease?

Alzheimer's disease is the cause of most cases of dementia. It is a chronic neurodegenerative disease. In America, the prevalence is less than 2% of the population under age 74, 19% in those aged 75 to 84, and 42% over age 84. Twin studies have shown a strong genetic component. Apolipoprotein E4 (APOE4) is one genetic risk factor. It is a protein found on lipoprotein particles carrying triglycerides and cholesterol in the blood. There are three versions of the protein, APOE2, APOE3, and APOE4. People who inherit only one APOE4 from their mother or father have a 3-fold increase in risk while those who inherit APOE4 from both parents have up to 15 times the risk of those without APOE4. Somewhere between 40 and 80% of those with Alzheimer's have at least one APOE4 gene.

**Here are the most important potentially modifiable risk factors for dementia:**

- Less education (1.6-fold increase in risk)
- Hypertension (1.6-fold)
- Obesity (1.6-fold)
- Hearing loss (1.9-fold)
- Smoking (1.6-fold)
- Depression (1.9-fold)
- Physical inactivity (1.4-fold)
- Social isolation (1.6-fold)
- Diabetes (1.5-fold)

**In terms of prevention, the following have been shown to be beneficial:**

- Learning a second language or a musical instrument
- Remaining intellectually active
- Social interactions
- Physical activity
- Mediterranean-style diet or other diet low in saturated fats and simple carbohydrates

The following pages are a self-administered test developed by Ohio State University to screen for early signs of Alzheimer's disease.

# How Well Are You Thinking?

Please complete this form in ink without the assistance of others

## Personal Information:

Name _____

Birth Date ____/____/____          I am a ...    Man    Woman

How far did you get in school?_____

I am ...    Asian        Black        Hispanic        White        Other

Have you had any problems with memory or thinking?

Yes                    Only Occasionally                    No

Have you had any blood relatives that have had problems
with memory or thinking?          Yes              No

Do you have balance problems?    Yes              No

If yes, do you know the cause?                    No
Yes (specify reason) _____

Have you ever had a major stroke?        Yes        No

A minor or mini-stroke?                  Yes        No

Do you currently feel sad or depressed?

Yes                    Only Occasionally                    No

Have you had any change in your personality?    No
Yes (specify changes) _____

Do you have more difficulties doing everyday activities
due to thinking problems?              Yes        No

Continue on next page →

106

1) What is today's date? (from memory - no looking!)
Month_____ Day_____ Year_____

2) Name the following pictures (don't worry about spelling)

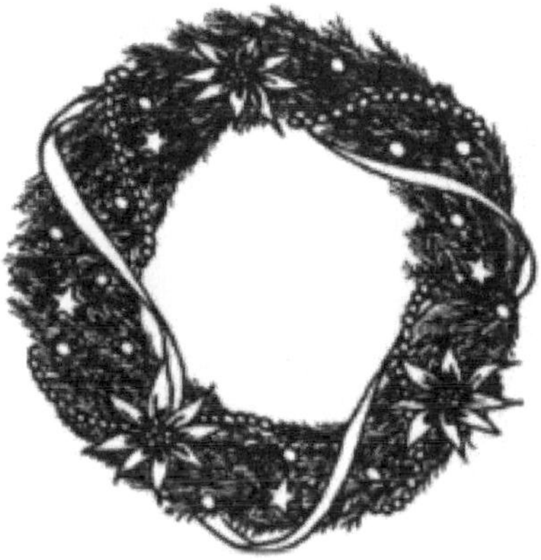

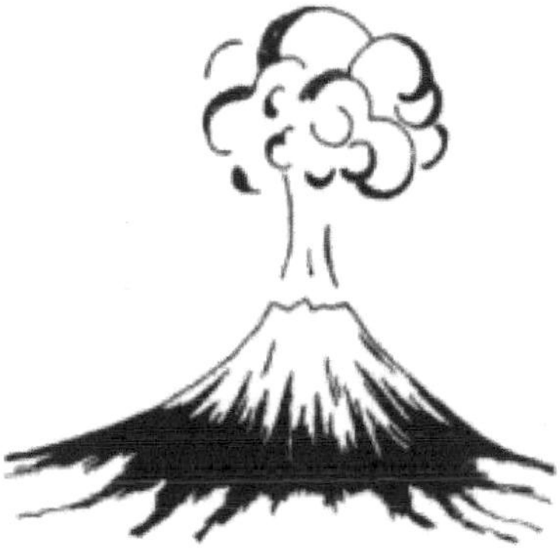

_____          _____

3) How are a watch and a ruler similar? Write down how
they are alike. They both ... _____

_____

_____

4) How many nickles are in 60 cents? _____

5) You are buying $13.45 of groceries. How much change
would you get back from $20? _____

Continue on next page →

6) Memorize these instructions, but do not do now:

After completing this entire test, write "I am done" on the blank line on the last page.

### Drawing Questions:

7) Copy this picture:

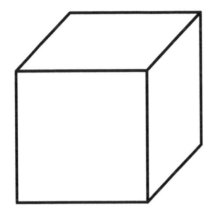

8) Draw a clock face and place in the numbers

Position the hands for 5 minutes after 11 o'clock

Label your clocks long hand "L" and short hand "S"

Continue on next page ➔

9) Write down the names of 12 different animals
(don't worry about spelling)

_____    _____    _____

_____    _____    _____

_____    _____    _____

_____    _____    _____

Review this example (this first one is done for you) then
complete the exersize yourself below. Draw a line from one
circle to another starting at 1 and alternating between numbers
and letters (1 to A to 2 to B to 3 to C).

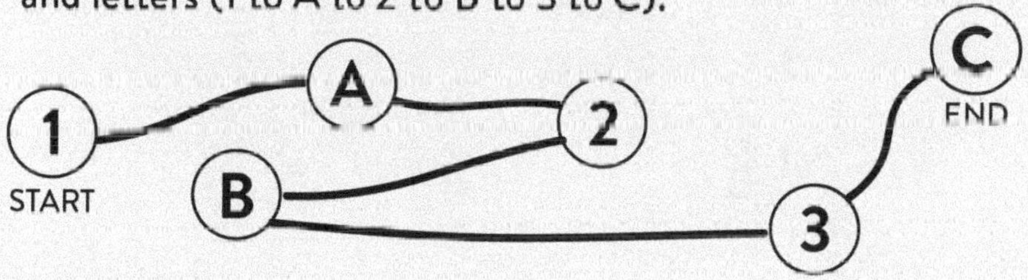

10) Now do it yourself here:

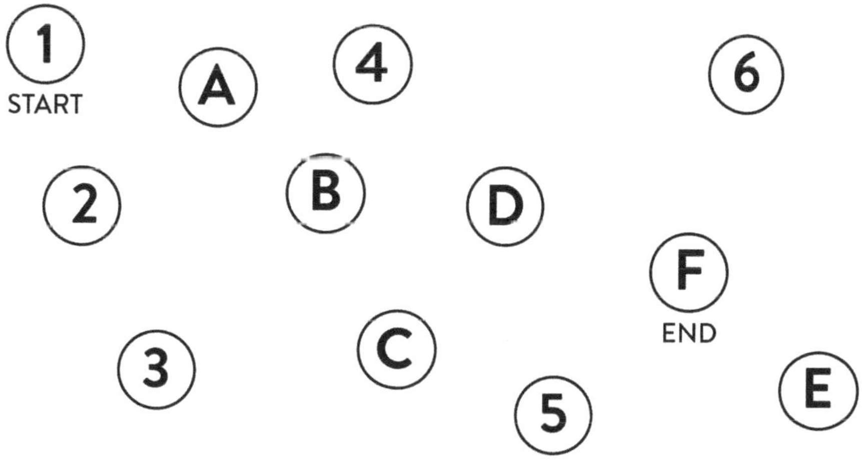

Continue on next page →

Review this example (this first one is done for you) then complete the exersize yourself below.

- Begin with 1 triangle and 1 square
- Move 2 lines (marked with an x)
- Make 2 squares and no triangle
- Each line must be part of a complete square (no extra lines)

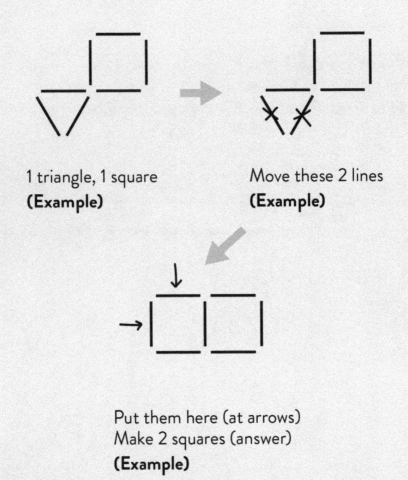

1 triangle, 1 square
**(Example)**

Move these 2 lines
**(Example)**

Put them here (at arrows)
Make 2 squares (answer)
**(Example)**

Continue on next page →

Now do it yourself here:

- Begin with 2 triangles and 2 squares
- Move 4 lines (mark which ones with an x)
- Make 4 squares and no triangle
- Each line must be part of a complete square (no extra lines)

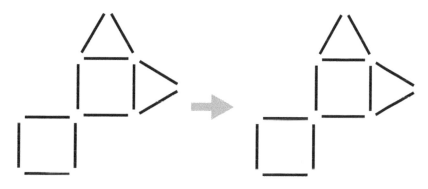

2 triangle, 2 square

Mark 4 lines to move with an X

Draw answer here

12) Have you finished? _____

End of Test

# How to Score

The first section "Personal Information" is not scored. It is designed to help one observe and reflect on memory function and motor skills.

The numbered questions are scored as follows:

**1) Month**
| Correct | 1 |
| Incorrect | 0 |

_____ points

**1) Date**
| Exact | 2 |
| +/- 3 days | 1 |
| Anything else | 0 |

_____ points

**1) Year**
| Correct | 1 |
| Incorrect | 0 |

_____ points

**2) Picture Naming**
| Wreath and volcano | 2 |
| One correct | 1 |
| Neither | 0 |

_____ points

**3) Similarities**
| Abstract (e.g. "they measure") | 2 |
| Concrete (e.g. "they have numbers) | 1 |
| All else | 0 |

_____ points

**4) Nickles**
| Answer: 12 | 1 |
| Anything else | 0 |

_____ points

**5) Change**
| Answer: $6.55 | 1 |
| Anything else | 0 |

_____ points

Continue on next page →

**6) Change**   Points given below in question 12

**7) 3D Box**

| | |
|---|---|
| 3D shape with parallel lines | 2 |
| 3D shape but lines more than 10 degrees from parallel | 1 |
| Anything else | 0 |

_____ points

**8) Clock**

| | |
|---|---|
| 4 of 4 correct | 2 |
| 3 of 4 (one must be hand positions) | 1 |
| <2 or incorrect hand positions | 0 |

_____ points

**4 Components:**
1) Clock face
2) Clock numbers (order & location)
3) Hand Positions
4) Hand Size (actual or properly labeled)

**9) Animals**

| | |
|---|---|
| 12 different animals | 2 |
| 10 or 11 | 1 |
| 9 or fewer | 0 |

_____ points

**10) Path**

| | |
|---|---|
| Perfect or self-corrected errors | 2 |
| 1 or 2 errors | 1 |
| More than 2 errors | 0 |

_____ points

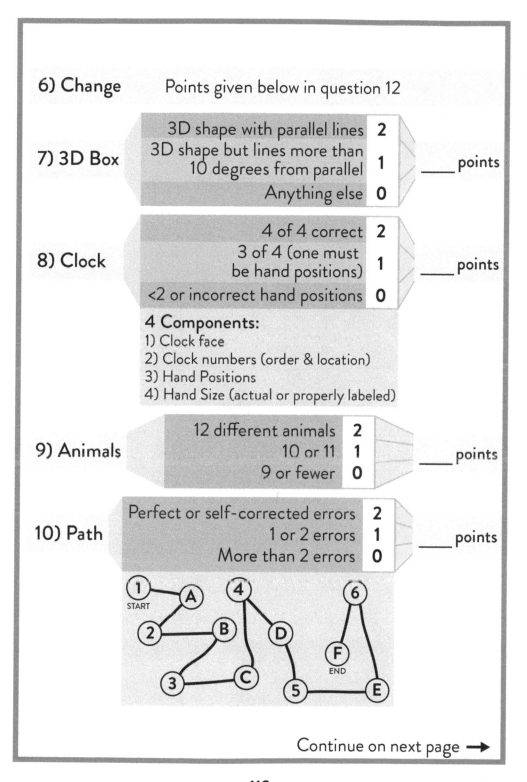

Continue on next page →

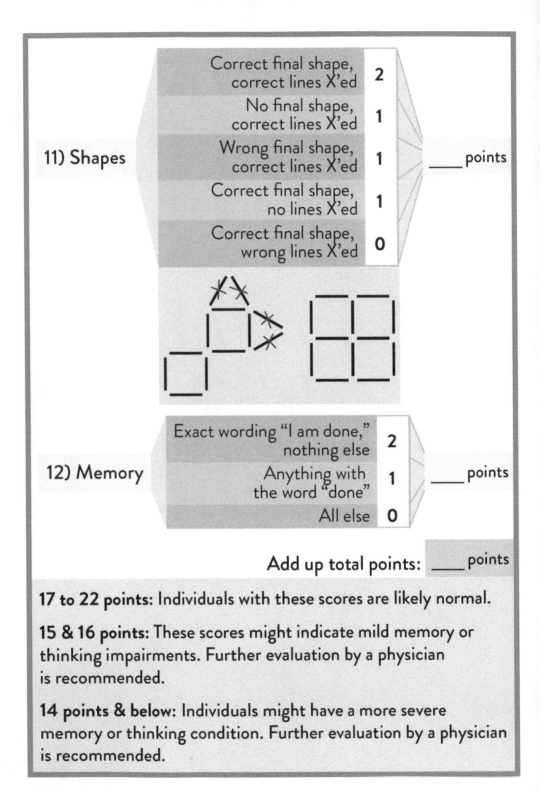

| 11) Shapes | Correct final shape, correct lines X'ed | 2 | \_\_\_\_ points |
| | No final shape, correct lines X'ed | 1 | |
| | Wrong final shape, correct lines X'ed | 1 | |
| | Correct final shape, no lines X'ed | 1 | |
| | Correct final shape, wrong lines X'ed | 0 | |

| 12) Memory | Exact wording "I am done," nothing else | 2 | \_\_\_\_ points |
| | Anything with the word "done" | 1 | |
| | All else | 0 | |

Add up total points: \_\_\_\_ points

**17 to 22 points:** Individuals with these scores are likely normal.

**15 & 16 points:** These scores might indicate mild memory or thinking impairments. Further evaluation by a physician is recommended.

**14 points & below:** Individuals might have a more severe memory or thinking condition. Further evaluation by a physician is recommended.

# Am I suffering from depression or anxiety?

Modern society, with its complexity and competitiveness, is a breeding ground for chronic stress. The stress response involves mobilization of various hormones and neurotransmitters, including adrenaline, noradrenaline and cortisol. These hormones are very useful in situations that require an immediate response to a dangerous situation or a focused response to an important task. But chronic stress is associated with chronic anxiety and depression. These can ultimately affect the immune system and make us more susceptible to chronic diseases.

A simple test, shown on the next page can help you quantify your levels of anxiety and depression.

# Mental Well Being

Give an immediate response to each question that best describes your current feelings. Do not think too long about your answers. Fill in the number of points in the circle or square.

**I feel tense or "wound up"**

| | |
|---|---|
| Most of the time | 3 |
| From time to time | 1 |
| A lot of the time | 2 |
| Not at all | 0 |

☐ points

**I still enjoy the things I used to enjoy**

| | |
|---|---|
| Definitely as much | 0 |
| Not quite so much | 1 |
| Only a little | 2 |
| Hardly at all | 3 |

◯ points

**I get a sort of frightened feeling as if something aweful is about to happen**

| | |
|---|---|
| Very definitely and quite bad | 3 |
| I do, but not too bad | 2 |
| A little but it doesnt worry me | 1 |
| Not at all | 0 |

☐ points

**I can laugh and see the fun side of things**

| | |
|---|---|
| As much as I always could | 0 |
| Not quite so much now | 1 |
| Definitely not so much now | 2 |
| Not at all | 3 |

◯ points

**Worrying thoughts go through my mind**

| | |
|---|---|
| A great deal of the time | 3 |
| A lot of the time | 2 |
| From time to time | 1 |
| Only occasionally | 0 |

☐ points

**I feel cheerful**

| | |
|---|---|
| Not at all | 3 |
| Not often | 2 |
| Sometimes | 1 |
| Most of the time | 0 |

◯ points

Continue on next page →

| I can sit at ease and feel relaxed | Definitely | 0 | | |
| | Usually | 1 | | |
| | Not often | 2 | ☐ | points |
| | Not at all | 3 | | |

| I feel as if I am slowed down | Nearly all the time | 3 | | |
| | Very often | 2 | | |
| | Sometimes | 1 | ◯ | points |
| | Not at all | 0 | | |

| I get a sort of frightened feeling like "butterflies" in my stomach | Not at all | 0 | | |
| | Occasionally | 1 | | |
| | Quite often | 2 | ☐ | points |
| | Very often | 3 | | |

| I have lost interest in my appearance | Definitely | 3 | | |
| | I don't take as much care as I should | 2 | | |
| | I may not take quite as much care | 1 | ◯ | points |
| | I take just as much care as ever | 0 | | |

| I feel restless as I have to be on the move | Very much indeed | 3 | | |
| | Quite a lot | 2 | | |
| | Not very much | 1 | ☐ | points |
| | Not at all | 0 | | |

| I look forward with enjoyment to things | As much as I ever did | 0 | | |
| | Rather less than I used to | 1 | | |
| | Definitely less than I used to | 2 | ◯ | points |
| | Hardly at all | 3 | | |

| I get sudden feelings of panic | Very often | 3 | | |
| | Quite often | 2 | | |
| | Not very often | 1 | ☐ | points |
| | Not at all | 0 | | |

Continue on next page →

| I can enjoy a good book or TV program | Often | 0 | |
|---|---|---|---|
| | Quite often | 1 | |
| | Not very often | 2 | ◯ points |
| | Very seldom | 3 | |

Add up total points for the circles and the squares:

Total ◯ points     Total ☐ points

**"Square" questions have to do with anxiety, while "Circle" questions have to do with happiness or depression.**
It is normal to feel a mixture of anxiety, happiness and sadness; however, if anxiety or depression are dominating your emotions they can cause problems which should be addressed by your doctor.

**14 to 21 points in "Circle" or "Square" individually**
Anxiety or depression is taking frequent and persistent toll. You should speak to your doctor.

**More than 20 points adding "Circle" and "Square" together**
Your feelings of anxiousness or sadness are impinging on your ability to enjoy life. You should talk to you doctor.

Another questionnaire that we utilize (found on the following pages) helps identify clients experiencing excessive amounts of stress.

# Perceived Stress Scale

The questions in this scale ask you about your feelings and thoughts **during the last month.** In each case, you will be asked to indicate how often you felt or thought a certain way.

| **0** | **1** | 2 | **3** | **4** |
|---|---|---|---|---|
| Never | Almost Never | Sometimes | Fairly Often | Very Often |

In the last month, how often have you been upset because of something that happened unexpectedly?  ☐ points

In the last month, how often have you felt that you were unable to control the important things in your life?  ☐ points

In the last month, how often have you felt nervous and "stressed"?  ☐ points

In the last month, how often have you felt confident about your ability to handle your personal problems?  ◯ points

In the last month, how often have you felt that things were going your way?  ◯ points

In the last month, how often have you felt that you could not cope with all the things that you had to do?  ☐ points

In the last month, how often have you been able to control irritations in your life?  ◯ points

Continue on next page →

In the last month, how often have you felt that you were on top of things? ◯ points

In the last month, how often have you been angered because of things that were outside of your control? ☐ points

In the last month, how often have you felt difficulties were piling up so high that you could not overcome them? ☐ points

Add up total points for the circles and the squares:

Total ◯ points        Total ☐ points

**"Square" questions are a measure of stress, while "Circle" questions are a measure of successful coping strategies for dealing with stress.**

**15 to 24 "Square" points:** You have many points of stress in your life that may be difficult to deal with all at once.

**10 to 16 "Circle" points:** Although you may have high levels of stress in your life, you feel fairly capable and confident that you can effectively deal with them.

**Subtract your "Circle" points from your "Square" points, if this number is greater than 10 then you are currently experience stress beyond your capacity to deal with.**

# How is my sleep?

Sleep deprivation is a common problem. Experts recommend 7-8 hours of sleep a night, but in America almost 40% of people get less than 7 hours. Performance levels for mental or physical activities show measurable declines after even one night with less than optimal sleep. People over age 45 have a two-fold increase in risk for heart attack or stroke when they sleep less than 6 hours a night. Blood pressure and pulse rate go up after 1 or 2 nights of inadequate sleep. Lack of sleep causes insulin resistance, which in turn increases risk for diabetes. Sleep deprivation increases levels of the hunger hormone- ghrelin, and decreases levels of the satiety hormone- leptin, thereby promoting obesity. The immune system suffers when we sleep less, lowering our resistance to infection, and decreasing the population of immune cells that destroy early cancers. Chronic sleep deprivation is associated with an increased risk for Alzheimer's disease, because it is during deep sleep that the amyloid deposits associated with the disease are effectively removed. Inadequate sleep adversely affects our emotional responses- and brain scans have shown that people with sleep deprivation have heightened activity in the amygdala- the part of our brain that is associated with anger and fear.

Sleep occurs in 90 minute cycles, passing from non-REM to REM sleep during the cycle, and going into the deepest sleep towards the end of the cycle. During non-REM (rapid eye movement) sleep, brain waves become synchronized and rhythmic, with hundreds of thousands of neurons working together, then falling silent, then beginning again. This activity indicates massive memory processing. During this phase, our bodies are completely calm, using very little energy. Blood pressure and pulse drop to low levels.

A very common cause of sleep deprivation is obstructive sleep apnea (OSA). This occurs when excess tissue in the upper airway obstructs air intake to the lungs. It is more common in people who are overweight but can also occur in thin people. Snoring is associated with sleep apnea, but not everyone who snores has the condition. People with OSA experience repeated episodes of airway closure during the night. This causes oxygen levels in the blood to drop. This in turn can have many adverse effects, including excessive daytime fatigue, high blood pressure, increased risk for heart attacks, cardiac arrhythmias, and elevated blood sugar levels.

Another common cause of sleep disruption is shift work. In America, over 22 million people work evening or night shifts. Shift work disrupts the circadian rhythm, and is associated with many adverse outcomes, including increased risk for diabetes, obesity, cognitive function, and cardiovascular disease.

The sleep/wake cycle is just the most obvious example of a circadian rhythm. Light during the day, particularly blue light, suppresses melatonin secretion by the pineal gland in the brain. When the sun sets, melatonin secretion begins to rise. Melatonin is just one example of a molecule with a 24 hour cycle. In

# Mind the Clock

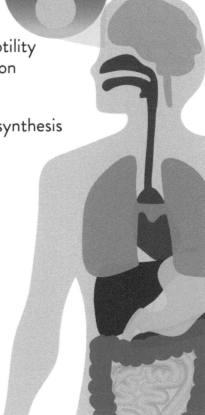

## Kidney
- Renal blood flow
- Potassium and sodium secretion

## Fat
- Lipid production and breakdown

## Gut
- Intestinal motility and absorption

## Liver
- Glycogen, cholesterol, and bile acid synthesis
- Glucose production
- Mitochondrial biogenesis

## Pancreas
- Insulin and glucagon secretion

## Muscle
- Fatty acid uptake
- Glycolytic and oxidative metabolism

## Cardiovascular Tissue
- Vascular tone and contractility
- Heart rate
- Blood pressure

fact, every cell in our body has the DNA machinery necessary for a circadian rhythm. Many molecules produced by our cells cycle up and down over a 24 hour period. The brain is able to synchronize all of these cellular circadian rhythms.

Because of circadian rhythms, we can map which bodily functions are most active at any particular time of the day-

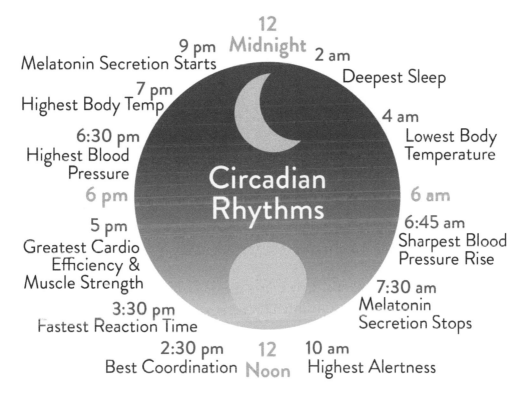

Also because of circadian rhythms, timing of food intake is very important for overall health. The circadian rhythm in liver cells programs them to be better at processing fats and sugars during the day. Research has shown that people who eat beyond a 12 hour daily window, particularly those who eat later in the evening, are more likely to develop insulin resistance, diabetes and other metabolic diseases. Eating and drinking alcohol after about 7pm also interferes with normal sleep patterns. Dr. Satchin Panda at the Salk Institute in La Jolla, CA has shown that time restricted feeding (TRF) in mice has many beneficial effects, including-

- Weight loss
- Improved blood glucose
- Reversal of fatty liver disease
- Improved blood lipids
- Lower levels of chronic inflammation
- Improved cardiovascular function

Many doctors are starting to recommend TRF to their patients. It is an easy program to initiate- simply count the hours from your first food or beverage intake to your last (not including water or calorie/caffeine-free beverages). A 12 hour eating window means you are fasting for 12 hours. A 10 hour eating window means you are fasting for 14 hours. A 8 hour eating window, such as from 9am to 5pm, indicates a 16 hour fasting period. The longer the fasting period, the greater the benefits.

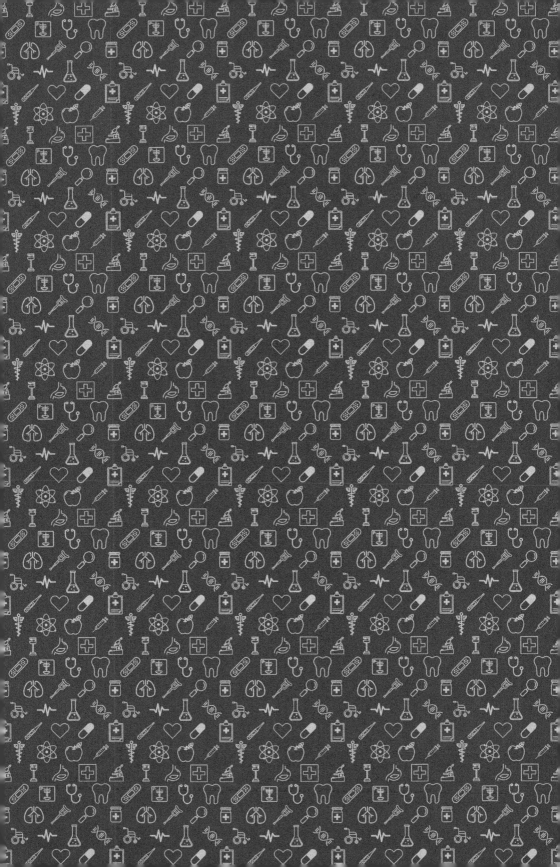

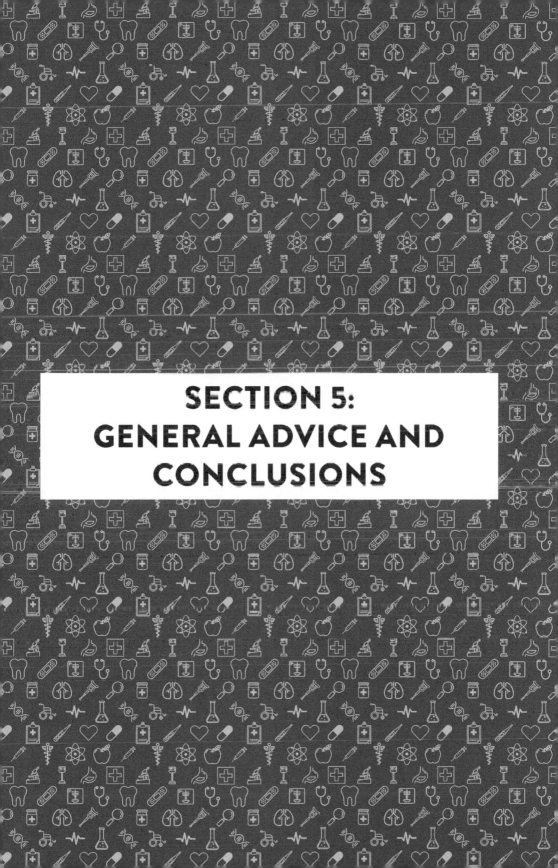

# SECTION 5:
# GENERAL ADVICE AND CONCLUSIONS

# How is my diet?

Dietary guidelines are typically created by scientific or government organizations. They review many lines of evidence and then create a set of recommendations that are considered suitable for the target population. For example, the Institute of Medicine releases its dietary guidelines for Americans every 5 years. The American Heart Association also has a set of dietary guidelines, meant to reduce risk for cardiovascular disease.

The problem with dietary guidelines is that they reduce nutrition to formulaic principles for large populations, and do not address the differences that exist between individuals concerning food preferences and genetic variability in food metabolism.

Nevertheless, many studies now support the beneficial effects of the Mediterranean diet. This is a diet that has been shown to reduce risk for many chronic diseases. It can be varied depending on individual preference and individual food tolerances (i.e. Not all people can tolerate a high intake of grains or a high intake of legumes).

The standard tool for assessing how closely someone's diet approximates the Mediterranean diet contains 147 items concerning food intake. This tool has been used in the large outcome studies that have shown a clear correlation between adherence to the diet and lower risk for cardiovascular disease. For our purposes, a much smaller set of questions is able to approximate the more comprehensive assessment and can give you a good idea about how closely your diet comes to being a Mediterranean diet.

In addition to scoring nutritional habits, this tool also has several questions that address other components of the Mediterranean lifestyle. It is good to remember that food is eaten within the context of a whole way of life. The Mediterranean lifestyle encompasses social interactions and daily activity levels. How much walking do you do? How often do you enjoy the company of others?

Overall, the Mediterranean lifestyle in conducive to a lower level of chronic stress and to a higher appreciation of the importance of things other than money and success.

The following pages contain an assessment tool. Each item is scored as a 0 or a 1. The highest score is 28. The higher your score, the closer your lifestyle is to the Mediterranean lifestyle. It is important to also remember that a healthy lifestyle does not depend on obsessively focusing on a limited number of rules. If you really like eating 1 or 2 eggs everyday, that does not mean you are necessarily adversely affecting your overall health. Yes, eggs do contain a significant amount of cholesterol, but that does not mean that they will significantly raise your serum cholesterol level (it depends on your genetics for cholesterol absorption across the intestinal wall, and many other aspects of cholesterol metabolism in the liver). In fact, eggs have also been shown to raise HDL cholesterol, which is protective for heart disease. Eggs also contain many other valuable nutrients, such as B vitamins (especially B12), lutein and zeaxanthin (eye health), vitamin A (eye health), and high quality protein.

It's also important to remember that there are other types of diets that can be quite healthy. An excellent book entitled The Blue Zones Solution describes the diets of 5 long-lived groups of people (Ikaria, Greece; Okinawa, Japan; Sardinia, Italy; Loma Linda, California; and Nicoya Peninsula, Costa Rica). Each group has its own specific set of foods, culturally determined, yet equally protective. Also, each group has a lifestyle that includes plenty of activity throughout the day, adequate sleep, and strong social bonds.

# Mediterranean Lifestyle

How many servings of pastries do you consume each week?

| | |
|---|---|
| 2 or fewer/week | 1 |
| More than 2/week | 0 |

_____ points

How many servings of red meat do you consume each week?

| | |
|---|---|
| 2 or fewer/week | 1 |
| More than 2/week | 0 |

_____ points

How many servings of processed meat do you consume each week?

| | |
|---|---|
| 1 or fewer/week | 1 |
| More than 1/week | 0 |

_____ points

How many eggs do you consume each week?

| | |
|---|---|
| 2-4/week | 1 |
| Anything else | 0 |

_____ points

How many servings of legumes do you consume each week?

| | |
|---|---|
| 2 or more/week | 1 |
| Fewer than 2/week | 0 |

_____ points

How many servings of white meat do you consume each week?

| | |
|---|---|
| About 2/week | 1 |
| Anything else | 0 |

_____ points

How many servings of fish or seafood do you consume each week?

| | |
|---|---|
| 2 or more/week | 1 |
| Fewer than 2/week | 0 |

_____ points

How many potatoes do you consume each week?

| | |
|---|---|
| 3 or fewer/week | 1 |
| More than 3/week | 0 |

_____ points

Continue on next page →

# Mediterranean Lifestyle

How many low-fat dairy products do you consume each day?

About 2/day **1**
Anything else **0**

_____ points

How many nuts and olives do you consume each day?

1 to 2 (or more)/day **1**
None **0**

_____ points

How many times do you use herbs for cooking each day? (onion, garlic, etc)

1 or more/day **1**
None **0**

_____ points

How many pieces of fruit do you consume each day?

3-6 or more/day **1**
Fewer than 3/day **0**

_____ points

How many servings of vegetables do you consume each day?

2 or more/day **1**
Fewer than 2/day **0**

_____ points

How many tablespoons of olive oil do you consume each day?

3 or more/day **1**
Fewer than 3/day **0**

_____ points

How many servings of whole grains do you consume each day?

2-4/day **1**
Fewer than 2/day **0**

_____ points

How many cups of water or tea do you drink each day?

At least 6 cups/day **1**
Less than 6 cups/day **0**

_____ points

Continue on next page →

# Mediterranean Lifestyle

| Do you drink wine at mealtime every day? | 0-2 servings/day | 1 | |
| | 3 or more/day | 0 | _____ points |

| Do you limit adding salt to your meals? | Yes | 1 | |
| | No | 0 | _____ points |

| Do you usually choose whole grain products? | Yes | 1 | |
| | No | 0 | _____ points |

| How many snacks do you have each week? (chips, popcorn, etc) | 2 or fewer/week | 1 | |
| | More than 2/week | 0 | _____ points |

| Do you usually limit nibbling between meals? | Yes | 1 | |
| | No | 0 | _____ points |

| Do you limit your intake of sugary beverages? | Yes | 1 | |
| | No | 0 | _____ points |

| Do you engage in physical activity? (150 min/week or 30 min/day or more) | Yes | 1 | |
| | No | 0 | _____ points |

| Do you take naps? | Yes | 1 | |
| | No | 0 | _____ points |

| How many hours of sleep do you get each night? (weekdays) | 6-9 hours/night | 1 | |
| | Anything else | 0 | _____ points |

Continue on next page →

# Mediterranean Lifestyle

| How many hours do you spend watching TV each day? (weekdays) | 1 hour or less/day | **1** | _____ points |
| More than 1 hr/day | **0** |

| How many hours do you spend with friends during your freetime (weekend) | 2 or more hrs/week | **1** | _____ points |
| Less than 2 hrs/week | **0** |

| How many hours do you practice team sports each week? | 2 or more/week | **1** | _____ points |
| Less than 2/week | **0** |

Add up total points: _____ points

**There are a maximum of 28 points.** As noted above, this is just one of many healthy diet and lifestyle guides. If you scored between **18 and 28 points** you are likely leading a very healthy lifestyle. If you scored less than **14 points** you should consider incorporating some of these practices into your life.

# What health screenings should I consider if I am over 40?

The best source for this information is the US preventive Services Task Force (USPSTF). USPTF is made up of 16 experts from many fields who serve on a voluntary basis for 4 year terms. The members are appointed by the Director of the Agency for Healthcare Research and Quality (AHRQ). AHRQ has been authorized by the US Congress to provide ongoing research and recommendations concerning preventive care for Americans. The following are the only screenings currently recommended.

## Screening for aortic aneurysm

- Recommend to men 65-75 years old who have ever smoked- one time screening with ultrasound
- Offer to men 65-75 who have never smoked
- Evidence not sufficient for women 65-74 who have ever smoked
- Screening not recommended for women 65-74 who have never smoked

## Screening for abnormal blood glucose

- Men and women 40-70 who are overweight or obese
- Earlier and/or more intensive screening for higher risk groups-
- History of gestational diabetes
- Polycystic ovarian disease
- Strong family history
- American Indian, Latino, southeast Asian, African-American, some others

# Breast cancer screening

- Women aged 40-49
  - » *If average risk, then individualized decision based on patient's understanding of higher number of false-positives leading to unnecessary biopsies, and higher number of diagnoses for non-life threatening cancers (over diagnosis)*
  - » *If 1st degree relative with breast cancer, then more justification for early screening*
- Women aged 50-74
  - » *Biennial screening recommended*
- Women aged 75 and over
  - » *Evidence insufficient for recommendation to screen*

# Cervical cancer screening

- Women aged 25 to 65
  - » *PAP smear every 3 years*
- Women aged 30 to 65 who wish less frequent screening
  - » *PAP smear plus HPV (human papilloma virus) testing every 5 years*

# Colorectal cancer screening

- Colonoscopy every 10 years from age 50 to 75
  - » *Period between screenings determined by findings at screening*
- Colonoscopy for those aged 76 to 85
  - » *Individual decision*
  - » *Best for those who are healthy enough to undergo treatment if cancer found and to benefit from treatment*
  - » *Those who have never been screened previously are more likely to benefit*
- Fecal occult blood test (FOBT or fecal immunochemical test (FIT) every year from age 50 to 75
  - » *Can be done at home*
  - » *FIT more accurate than FOBT*

# Screening for depression

- Recommended for the general adult population
  - » *Systems should be in place to insure adequate diagnosis, treatment and follow-up*

## Screening for high blood pressure

- Periodic screening is recommended for all adults aged 18 and older

## Screening for lung cancer

- Recommended to have yearly low dose computed tomography (CT scan) if-
  - » *Between ages 55 to 80*
  - » *30 or greater pack-years of smoking (a pack-year is one pack per day for a year)*
  - » *Currently smokes or has quit within the past 15 years*
- Screening should be discontinued once a person has not smoked for 15 years or has another health problem that substantially reduces life-expectancy

## Screening for obesity

- Screen all adults for obesity
  - » *If BMI 30 or greater-*
  - » *Refer for intensive behavioral interventions*

# Do I have a proactive relationship with my doctors?

Most doctors spend 5 to 15 minutes in face to face contact during an outpatient visit. To prepare for this brief encounter, you should be as educated as possible on the issues that are going to be discussed. If you are seeing the doctor for the first time, provide him/her with a description of your past medical history, including significant illnesses, surgeries and hospitalizations. Also have a list of your medications, doses and schedules. Results of labs and imaging studies are also very important to provide a complete picture of your medical history and to avoid duplicate testing. Finally, make sure to inform your physician of any diseases or conditions in your family history.

You should also be able to discuss your current condition. Are you experiencing any symptoms of concern? Are you aware of the ongoing indications for the medications you are taking? Are you experiencing any potentially adverse effects from the medications?

Here is a list of the narrative components that may be included in a doctor visit:
• Preventive care- includes items such as risk factor profile for cardiovascular disease, appropriate cancer screening tests, diabetes screening if appropriate, weight counseling, substance abuse counseling and healthy lifestyle counseling.
• Mental well-being discussion- to assess for excessive stress, anxiety or depression.
• Questions about current medical problems- This might include medication review, symptom review, diagnostic test review, prognosis, etc.
• Questions about any new conditions or symptoms.
• Physical exam- weight, blood pressure, pulse, heart and lung exam, extremities and skin condition, with other components of the exam directed towards specific symptoms, such as sore throat, ear pain, joint pain, neurological symptoms, gastrointestinal symptoms, etc.

- List of medical problems and status of each. Plan of action for each medical problem.
- Follow-up plan.

Be prepared for your doctor visits. Make sure that your visit covered all of your current concerns, but also be aware of the time constraints on physicians. Make sure you have a good rapport with your doctor, and that he or she knows how to listen. Try to list the goals for your visit, and make your physician aware of these goals at the beginning of the encounter. If you do not feel comfortable with your doctor, you should consider a change. A doctor should not just be a technician. A good doctor will make you feel at ease, will encourage you to share your concerns, and will provide you with up to date information on all the options available for your treatment.

# How can I use digital tools to improve my health?

Smartphones and digital watches are rapidly evolving in their capabilities to help us improve our lifestyles. This brief overview demonstrates how the iPhone and AppleWatch can be used to track activity, nutrition and even sleep. Many other options are also available.

## Exercise and activity

The iPhone Health app provides a handy place to store health data. When used with the AppleWatch, you can track three components of an active lifestyle called Move, Exercise and Stand. Data can be looked at as a summary for 24 hours or broken down by hour. You can choose a face for the AppleWatch that shows three coloured circles, each representing one component of activity. The red circle indicates the number of calories burned in movement/day, with the default goal 600 calories. The red circle gradually grows as calories are clocked, until the completed circle indicates goal achievement. The yellow circle moves towards completion as the goal of 30 minutes of exercise is reached. The blue circle is linked to standing for at least 5 minutes per hour for at least 12 hours of the day.

All this information can keep you focused on fighting the health risks of a sedentary lifestyle. Prolonged inactivity, such as sitting for more than 1 or 2 hours at a time, increases the risk for diabetes and other obesity-related conditions.

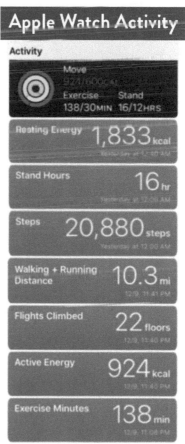

139

This is why the app calls attention to 3 separate components of an active lifestyle. Exercise is calculated as sustained cardio activity for at least 10 minute intervals. Movement on the other hand can be climbing stairs or walking from one place to another at work or in the home or at a store. Remembering to stand for at least 5 minutes at the end of an hour in a chair can dramatically reduce the adverse effects of sitting. The app also keeps track of daily steps. For optimal health, 10-15,000 steps should be walked each day.

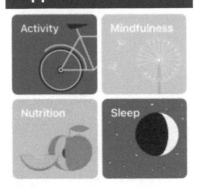

The Apple Health app also has sections on nutrition, mindfulness and sleep-

Each of these components can be linked to dozens of apps in the App Store. Many other companies, such as Fitbit, Garmin and Nokia offer wearables that perform similar functions to the AppleWatch.

# Is my symptom serious?

It can be very challenging to assess the importance of a symptom. How do you know if the symptom is a superficial and transitory problem or if it is linked to a more serious underlying condition? In this section we will list some common symptoms and give you some key insights into differentiating between a minor or potentially major health issue.

## Headache

Headaches that are severe should always be evaluated by your physician. Also headaches that are accompanied by other symptoms, such as visual changes, hearing loss, vertigo, or neurological signs in the arms or legs, should be medically evaluated. Mild to moderate headaches are very common, and usually are due to tension in the scalp muscles, eye strain, or other factors such as chronic stress.

## Cough

Coughs are triggered by an irritated airway. Upper airway irritation usually results in a dry cough, while lower airway irritation often results in a productive cough. Airways can be irritated by particulate matter in the air we breathe, or by infections, either viral or bacterial. Bronchial tubes can also be irritated by a tumor, or by fluid congestion in heart failure. Productive coughs, bloody coughs, or chronic coughs should always be investigated by a physician.

## Shortness of breath

Occurs when not enough oxygen is reaching organs and tissues to meet metabolic requirements. The medical term for this is dyspnea. Dyspnea increases respiratory rate in an effort to bring more oxygen to the alveoli (the sacs at the end of the bronchial tubes) where it diffuses into the blood stream. Dyspnea on exertion is normal when the level of exertion is moderate or greater. Dyspnea at rest or with mild exertion is abnormal and may indicate a serious problem with the heart or lungs. Dyspnea when lying down may indicate heart failure. Sudden onset of dyspnea with no associated cough could mean a pulmonary embolism (blood clot in the lungs). Dyspnea with a productive cough may be a pneumonia. Always seek medical help if you are experiencing new onset dyspnea.

## Chest pain

There are many potential causes for chest pain. If the pain is pressure-like or squeezing and occurs with exertion it may be angina (the pain associated with inadequate blood flow to the heart muscle). Angina can also be felt in the neck or left arm. Angina can also occur at rest. Typically angina only lasts a few minutes. Any squeezing-type pain should be evaluated by your doctor as soon as possible. Prolonged squeezing chest pain, especially if accompanied by dyspnea, sweating and nausea, could indicate a heart attack and requires immediate transfer to an emergency room in an ambulance. Chest pain related to inspiration could indicate inflammation in the lining around the lungs (pleura) or heart (pericardium). Less serious types of chest pain are often musculoskeletal, due to inflammation or injury to the chest wall, or gastrointestinal, due to reflux of stomach contents up into the esophagus.

## Abdominal pain

Severe abdominal pain that comes on suddenly should be evaluated immediately, as it could indicate a severe inflammation, such as appendicitis, cholecystitis (gall bladder inflammation), peritonitis (inflammation of the abdominal cavity), a perforated ulcer, or diverticulitis (inflammation of a diverticulum). Alternatively, it could indicate rupture of an aortic aneurysm, a potentially catastrophic event. Mild to moderate abdominal pain can occur with irritable bowel syndrome, gastritis, mild forms of diverticulitis, gallstones, gastroesophageal reflux disease, viral infections of the GI tract, and many other less common conditions.

## Palpitations

Most people experience occasional palpitations, often described as a skipped beat, a fluttering sensation, or abnormal pounding of the heart. The most common underlying cause for a skipped beat or a sudden extra forceful heartbeat is a premature beat. These are caused by groups of heart muscle cells that have the ability to depolarize spontaneously. Normally depolarization starts in the sinoatrial node at the top of the heart. Depolarization means the inside of the cell membrane becomes more positively charged. This wave of positive charge travels through specialized tissue from the sinoatrial node and triggers cardiac contraction. Premature depolarization can occur in clusters of cells in the upper or lower chambers of the heart (atria or ventricles). A premature depolarization originating in the upper chambers is called a premature atrial contraction (PAC), while one from the lower chambers is called a premature ventricular contraction (PVC). We all experience these occasionally, but when they occur frequently they may indicate an underlying cardiac problem, and should be reported to your physician. Excessive caffeine or alcohol intake, severe stress, and lack of sleep are common triggers for premature beats. Illicit drugs such as cocaine and amphetamines can also cause abnormal heartbeats. When palpitations are more sustained, they are often described as a suddenly racing heart, either in a regular or irregular pattern. If the heart rate goes extremely fast, then lightheadedness might develop, or even loss of consciousness. At rates over 200, the ventricles don't have time to completely fill before the next depolarization signal arrives, so cardiac output drops and the brain cannot function normally. Sudden onset of a racing heart may indicate a serious rhythm disturbance and should be medically evaluated.

## Lightheadedness

This symptom means the brain is not getting enough oxygen. It can occur when getting up too quickly, particularly if you have low blood pressure (normally or from too aggressive treatment for high blood pressure) or are dehydrated. It can also occur if the heart rate is too fast or too slow, and in disorders of the autonomic nervous system. If you are experiencing severe or prolonged lightheadedness you should seek medical help.

## Fatigue

This is one of the most common symptoms a doctor confronts. How then to distinguish fatigue with no underlying identifiable medical cause (due to boredom, mild sleep deprivation, poor diet, chronic stress, and many other lifestyle factors) from fatigue that indicates disease?  If you believe your fatigue is significantly impacting your ability to function normally and enjoy life, you should seek medical evaluation. Common problems that can cause fatigue include hypothyroidism, anemia, chronic fatigue syndrome, sleep apnea, bradycardia (slow heart rate) and moderate or severe depression.

# How good is my knowledge of the topics covered in this book?

## Case histories from Scripps Center of Executive Health Medical Director Dr. Scott Carstens

| Quiz Yourself |
|---|
| **Circle all that apply** |

### Case 1

45 year old male with strong family history of premature coronary artery disease

**1) Which of the following tests would be important to further assess his risk for heart attack?**

a. Blood lipids (cholesterol, triglycerides and lipoprotein particles)
b. Thyroid function
c. Blood pressure
d. Carotid ultrasound
e. Coronary calcium score

### Case 2

65 year old female with anxiety, insomnia and borderline high blood pressure

Continue on next page ➡

**2) Which of the following would be helpful for relieving anxiety and/or insomnia?**

a. 30 to 60 minutes of moderate exercise a day
b. Rewarding social interactions with friends and or community
c. Limiting television viewing to less than 2 hours/day
d. Avoiding excessive caffeine intake, especially after 3pm
e. Substituting herbal teas for sodas
f. Taking an appropriate dose of melatonin 1 hour before bedtime

**3) Which of the following would be least effective in treating borderline high blood pressure?**

a. A low dose of a calcium channel blocker
b. Losing weight if overweight or obese
c. Eating a diet high in fruits and vegetables
d. Reducing sodium intake
e. Exercising on a regular basis

## Case 3

A 54 year old male with low back pain and cholesterol concerns

**4) Which of the following signs would indicate a potentially dangerous back condition?**

a. Symptoms only occurring when wife asks patient to do household fix-up project
b. Symptoms occur with excessive exercise, such as training for a marathon
c. Symptoms occur when bending over to pick up a box
d. Tingling and numbness in the right foot
e. Pain occurring immediately after acute trauma

Continue on next page →

**5) The patient's total cholesterol is 260mg/dL. Which of the following lipid panel results are of concern?**

a. Triglycerides 86mg/dL
b. HDL cholesterol 78mg/dL
c. LDL cholesterol 165mg/dL

**6) What other factors would be important in deciding whether to treat the LDL cholesterol?**

a. Family history of coronary artery disease
b. Prior history of "mild" heart attack
c. History of asthma
d. Obesity
e. Presence of high blood pressure
f. Stressful job

## Case 4

62 year old male with high blood pressure

**7) The patient's blood pressure was 160/80. He is on three blood pressure medications. What should be his blood pressure goal?**

a. Less than 160/85
b. Less than 150/85
c. Less than 140/80
d. Less than 130/80

Continue on next page →

8) This patient also had a triglyceride level of 426. Which of the following statements is true?

a. High triglyceride level is defined as 200-500
b. Triglycerides are carried in VLDL particles
c. Omega-3 fish oil capsules can lower triglycerides
d. High triglycerides are part of the metabolic syndrome
e. High triglycerides are a risk factor for diabetes

## Case 5

43 year old female who gets up at 4am everyday and must balance responsibilities of being a mother, wife and marketing director job

9) Which of the following conditions could be related to inadequate sleep?

a. High blood pressure
b. Overweight
c. Anxiety
d. Diabetes
e. Increased risk for heart attack
f. Increased risk for cancer
g. Increased risk for Alzheimer's disease

## Case 6

42 year old male with sleep apnea and gastroesophageal reflux (GERD)

Continue on next page →

## 10) Which of the following are associated with sleep apnea?

a. Cardiac arrhythmias
b. Overweight or obese status
c. Cigarette smoking
d. Caffeine intake
e. Snoring

## 11) Which of these statements are true about GERD?

a. There are no serious risks associated with this condition
b. Chocolate, coffee and alcohol can worsen symptoms
c. Elevating the head of the bed at night is not helpful for symptoms relief
d. Stopping to eat 2-3 hours before bedtime helps reduce symptoms
e. Weight loss can improve symptoms

**Answers:**

**1)** all except b
**2)** all
**3)** d
**4)** d and e
**5)** c
**6)** a, b and e
**7)** d
**8)** all
**9)** all
**10)** a, b and e
**11)** b, d and e

# What are the most important things I should be doing to prevent age-related chronic disease?

Death is inevitable, but there are different ways of dying. For so many people in America, death is the culmination of a gradual loss of health over several decades, as one chronic condition after another invades the body and diminishes quality of life. Surprisingly, genetics plays a relatively small role compared to lifestyle for most chronic diseases. A small percentage of people have significant enough genetic mutations that disease is inevitable regardless of lifestyle. For the rest of us, genetic tendencies may influence the effects of lifestyle decisions. Each of our genes has accumulated random changes over time. These changes may subtly affect the properties of the molecule coded by the gene. A gene related to blood pressure or obesity or triglyceride level may have dozens of variants. Some of these variants will lessen the likelihood of the associated medical condition and some will increase the likelihood.

For this reason, it is important that you understand which conditions you are more likely to develop so that you can proactively alter your lifestyle or begin a medication to remain healthy. Family medical history is one way of gaining insight into your risks. If you have a strong family history of heart disease you should discuss this with your physician. You may have a genetic predisposition for high blood pressure, diabetes, or lipid abnormalities that are associated with the premature onset of atherosclerosis. If there is a strong family history of cancer, you may be a candidate for genetic screening.

But regardless of your particular genetic makeup, there are certain behaviors that will greatly increase your likelihood of remaining healthy for as long as possible. Here is a list of the 11 best ways to avoid chronic disease:

## 1) Cultivate an active lifestyle
Exercise for 30-60 minutes a day, and during the rest of the day stand and

walk frequently. Avoid sitting for long periods of time. Make sure your exercise program is safe and fun for you.

## 2) Eat your meals within an 8-12 hour window each day

Have a healthy breakfast, and try to have your last food and beverage (other than water or herbal tea) by 6 or 7 in the evening. On the weekends you can cheat!

## 3) Cultivate strong social networks with people that have a positive influence on your life

Do not spend time with people that make you feel insecure, inadequate, or fearful. Avoid angry and unpleasant people. At work, learn how to deal with toxic personality types by remaining calm and confronting any kind of abuse with gentle resistance and rational rebuttal. Be fair and kind with all those around you.

## 4) Do not smoke or use tobacco

Do not smoke cigarettes or use other forms of tobacco such as snuff or chewing tobacco. Tobacco cause cancer, cardiovascular disease and chronic lung disease.

## 5) Cook meals at home as frequently as possible

Think of meal preparation as a pleasurable experience. Share your meals with friends and family. Use mealtimes as opportunities for relaxation and socialization.

## 6) Avoid processed foods as much as possible

A healthy diet consists primarily of natural fruits and vegetables, whole grains, legumes, healthy oils, such as olive, avocado, walnut, grapeseed and coconut oil (despite being high in saturated fat, coconut oil contains healthy medium chain triglycerides), nuts and seeds, and seafood. With this foundation, don't be afraid to enjoy other foods from time to time. Because we each have different genetic predispositions, some people can eat high cholesterol foods such as eggs with impunity. In fact, eggs and saturated fat are not that dangerous, especially in moderation and in the setting of an overall healthy diet. Processed meats are more dangerous than red meat. Do not snack excessively between meals. Above all, enjoy food! Do not feel guilty about eating some butter, ice cream, cheese or other "sinful" food from time to time.

## 7) Sleep 7-8 hours per night

## 8) Spend time outdoors in nature, as disconnected as possible from your electronic devices

## 9) Be selective with TV watching
Restrict viewing to no more than 2 hours on most days.

## 10) Cultivate relaxation techniques
From yoga to biofeedback, from mindfulness to meditation, there are many stress reduction techniques that can improve quality of life and overall health.

## 11) Use alcohol sparingly
1-2 drinks per day is safe for most people and lowers risk for cardiovascular disease. Larger quantities are associated with high blood pressure, liver disease and cancer.